The Journey Beyond Breast Cancer

FROM THE PERSONAL TO THE POLITICAL

Taking an Active Role in Prevention, Diagnosis, and Your Own Healing

VIRGINIA M. SOFFA

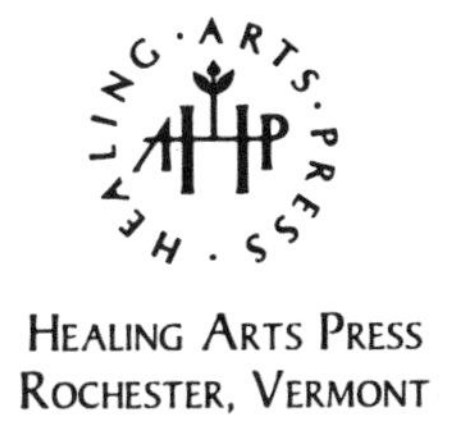

HEALING ARTS PRESS
ROCHESTER, VERMONT

Healing Arts Press
One Park Street
Rochester, Vermont 05767

Note to the reader: *This book is intended as an informational guide. The remedies, approaches, and techniques described herein are meant to supplement, and not to be a substitute for, professional medical care or treatment. They should not be used to treat a serious ailment without prior consultation with a qualified healthcare professional.*

Library of Congress Cataloging-in-Publication Data
Soffa, Virginia M., 1951–
The journey beyond breast cancer : from the personal to the political: taking an active role in prevention, diagnosis, and your own healing / Virginia M. Soffa.
p. cm.
Includes bibliographical references and index.
ISBN 0-89281-448-9
1. Soffa, Virginia M., 1951—Health. 2. Breast—Cancer—Patients—United States—Biography. 3. Breast—Cancer—Alternative treatment. I. Title.
RC280.B8S565 1992
362.1'969949'092—dc20
[B]
92-24188
CIP

Printed and bound in the United States

10 9 8 7 6 5 4 3 2 1

Text design by Bonnie Atwater and Virginia L. Scott

Healing Arts Press is a division of Inner Traditions International

Distributed to the book trade in the United States by American International Distribution Corporation (AIDC)

Distributed to the book trade in Canada by Publishers Group West (PGW), Montreal West, Quebec

Distributed to the health food trade in Canada by Alive Books, Toronto and Vancouver

Distributed to the book trade in the United Kingdom by Deep Books, London

Distributed to the book trade in Australia by Millennium Books, Newtown, N. S. W.

Distributed to the book trade in New Zealand by Tandem Press, Auckland, New Zealand

The Journey Beyond Breast Cancer

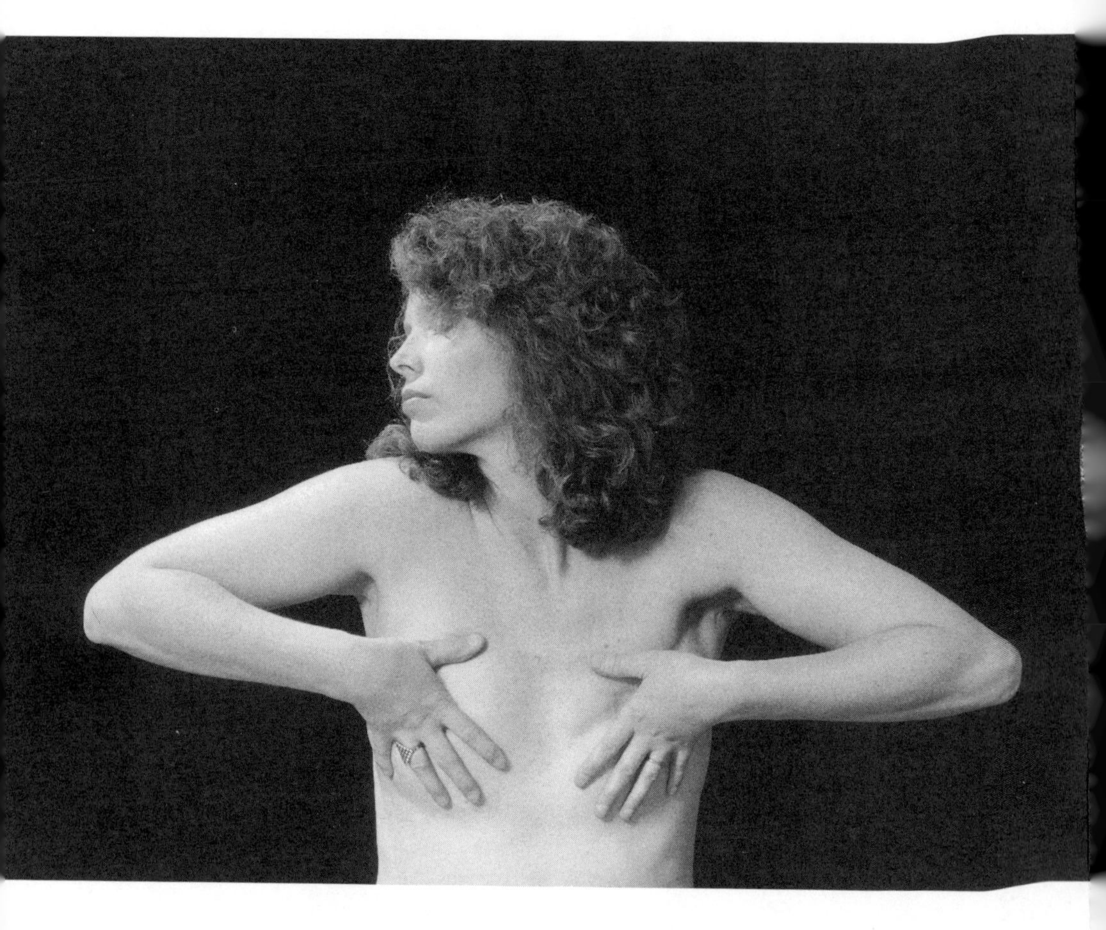

The Road Back—Self Portrait II
Susan B. Markisz, Riverdale, New York
Silver gelatin print, 8" x 10" framed to 16" x 20", 1991

The artwork and statements that appear throughout this book are from the "Healing Legacies" arts registry that was first exhibited at the U.S. House of Representatives Cannon Office Building Rotunda in October of 1993—National Breast Cancer Awareness Month.

I dedicate this book to:

All the women who die of breast cancer.
May they be remembered for the way they lived their lives.

All the women who have been diagnosed with breast cancer.
May you find purpose in this experience.

All who have been touched by breast cancer indirectly or directly.
May you find your role to help in some small way
put an end to this epidemic.

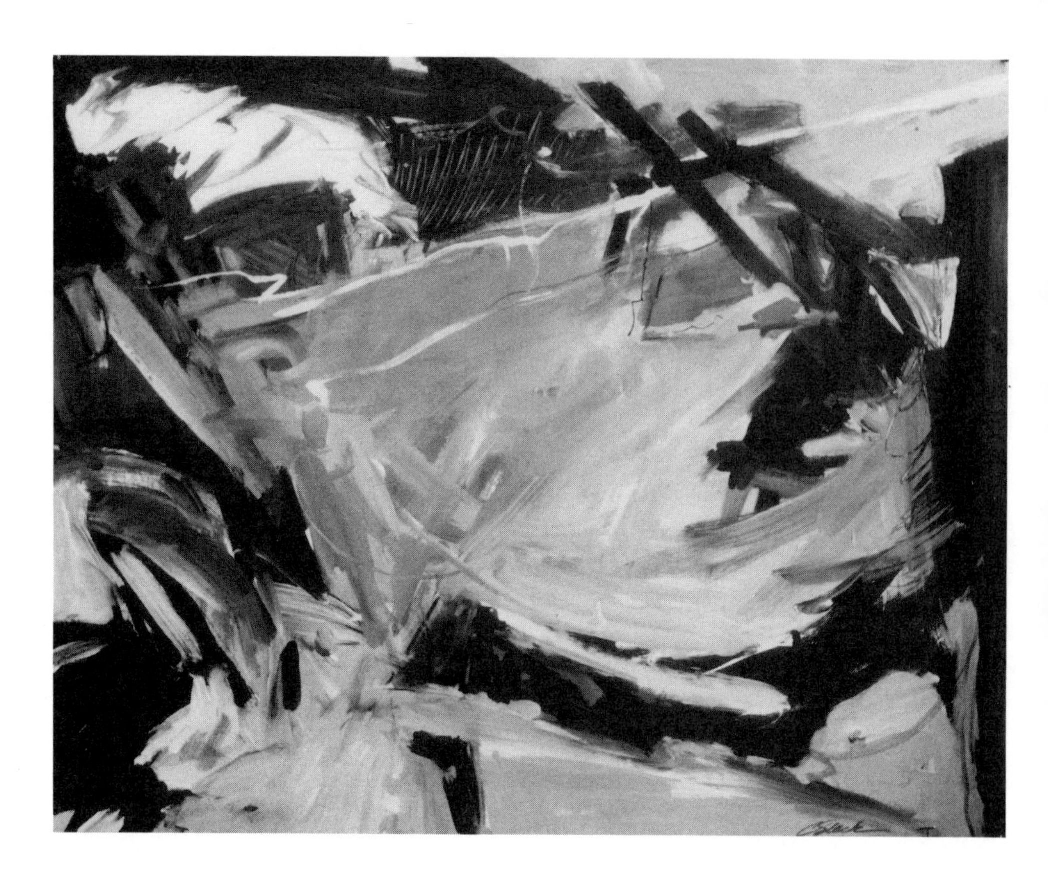

Love in the Rain
Connie Slack, Alexandria, Virginia
Acrylic on paper, 44" x 52", 1993

"Discovering that I have breast cancer has become a wake-up call for me. A call to be as honest as possible in my relationships and my communication. Painting is my purest form of communication and honesty of expression is a constant challenge for me to examine and reveal what is true for me through my paintings. The reality that pervades is one of joy for life's wonders as well as an acute sense of God's ever-present grace."

Contents

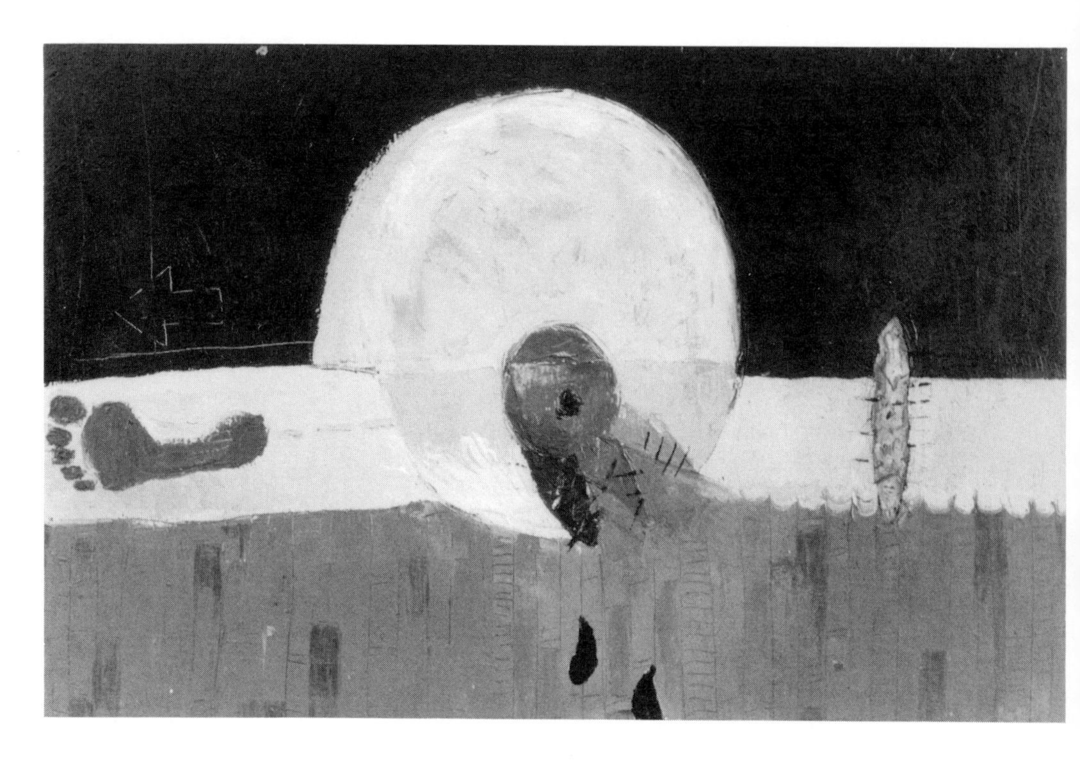

Weeping
Joan Thompson Kehrl, Rockville, Maryland
Oil on canvas, 24" x 36", 1993

*"*Weeping *has to do with the effect breast cancer has on some relationships. Often this can be as insidious as the tumor's effect on the body. Now in my mid-40s, I am planning on a long productive painting career and plenty of time to enjoy my two teenaged sons as they grow through life. Yet I can't ignore or deny the fact that breast cancer has had an effect on my life whose perimeters are still being defined."*

Acknowledgments

When I started this book I never imagined that it would take more than four years from inception to completion. There are therefore many people to recognize whom I came in contact with during this process. The task for me began with finding a writing support team: Jules Older, a writing instructor of unique proportions; K. K. Wilder, my writing coach; Pamela Polston, who is not only a true friend but on-call editor; and Barbara DuBois, who was a continuous source of inspiration. These people gave me the encouragement to put my thoughts to paper and helped me refine what I wrote so others could understand it.

My research process was facilitated by the unlimited use of the University of Vermont Medical School library, as well as friends and doctors who answered questions and sent me the latest articles contributing to the accuracy and currentness of what I was writing: Marcia Rhodes, a fellow survivor who was always on the outlook for what was new; Neal Barnard, M.D.; Wayne London, M.D.; Pat Bredenberg, Ph.D.; Susan Love, M.D.; David Eddy, M.D.; Taddy Dickerson, Ph.D.; Judith Karp, M.D., Special Assistant to the Director of the National Cancer Institute; and Teresa Squires, Statistical Information Specialist at the American Cancer Society.

I am eternally grateful to those that came to my aid during the writing process, offering whatever was needed at the moment: Sharon Batt, who reviewed my earliest manuscript and offered suggestions; Beverly Jacobson, who was an ever present inspiration; and Pat Winer and my research assistant Jennifer Wagner, who volunteered endless hours and long nights tracking down the details needed for all the footnotes.

This book would not contain the depth of experience it has were it not for my wholistic healing guides and teachers: Sahra Aschenbach, Blake Gould, Robin Hopps, Holly Pedrini, Arthur Makaris, Chun-Han Zhu,

Winston Lewis, Yogi Amrit Desai, Satyajit, Aviva, and Jesse Thompson.

Additionally there were the many women who were my friends and allies in pioneering the grassroots breast cancer movement, who worked with me to get the early political agenda on track: Ellen Crowley, Elenore Pred, Mary Jo Kahn, Sheila Swanson, and Susan Claymon.

I thank Vermont's congressional members and their staff members for working so closely with me on bringing about new legislation and awareness and enlightening me about how Washington politics works: Senator Patrick Leahy, Theresa Alberghini, Senator James Jeffords, Peter Caldwell, Vicki Caldera, Congressman Bernard Sanders, Katie Clarke, Jane Sanders, and Liz Gibbs-West. I also thank the four women who helped me organize the Breast Cancer Action Group: Barbara Scheuer, Billie Tudhope, Kathe Tiballi, and Pamela Polston, and all the artists who had the courage and determination to participate in the premier exhibit of "Healing Legacies: A Collection of Art and Writing by Women with Breast Cancer" at the U.S. House of Representatives Cannon Office Building Rotunda. Having their work in my book is an honor.

I hold a special appreciation for Leslie Colket, then managing editor at Inner Traditions, who read my proposal and saw its potential. I thank her for being more than an editor, but also sharing her friendship throughout the many months needed to organize the manuscript so that everyone could understand what I wanted to present. Thanks to Gretchen Gordon, Anna Chapman, and Jeanie Levitan for their close attention to detail as they proofread and sheparded along the manuscript to publication, and to Melinda Molin, M.D., for her medical review. And finally a depth of gratitude to my publisher Ehud Sperling, who always kept a careful eye on new findings reported in the *Wall Street Journal* and stayed committed to seeing this book published.

It is clear to me without the help of all these individuals, and some that I have no doubt missed mentioning, that this book would only be another great idea.

Introduction

This book is very frank, that is, I tell the hard truth about breast cancer. For this reason, it may not be what you want to hear, particularly if you're someone who only wants to be told stories about how to triumph over breast cancer. I have learned that every woman's experience is very different, and I respect every woman for the way she approaches her treatment and regains control over her life. That is why I offer this word of caution, because I don't want to be blamed for taking away anyone's hope. The fact is, the truth about breast cancer is a hard pill to swallow.

I was no different from the estimated 160,000[1] other American women who were diagnosed with breast cancer in 1989. I believed that the treatment and the survival rate for breast cancer had improved. I believed that it was important to have an annual physical exam and to periodically do my own breast self-exam (BSE). I believed everything the media were promoting about early detection being our best defense against breast cancer. That is, I believed it until it was my turn to hear that I had breast cancer.

That's when this myth began to unravel for me. I learned there is more to curing breast cancer than early detection and lumpectomy. I began to conduct my own investigation into the approaches of diagnosing and treating breast cancer. I started searching for the best path to restoring my health. And eventually I came to realize that breast cancer is not only a personal issue but also very much a feminist and political issue.

Since 1960, when the American Cancer Society began to track cancer deaths, more than a million men and women have died from breast cancer (less than 1 percent have been men). Today 1,758,000 women live with breast cancer as a chronic condition. Every woman over fifteen years old is at risk for getting breast cancer. In 1994, twenty-one women will be diagnosed with breast cancer every hour, and slightly over five women every hour will die from this cancer.

I was only thirty-eight years old when I found out that I had breast cancer. The surgeon removed a one-centimeter tumor by incisional biopsy to make the diagnosis. At this time, two different medical labs determined that the tissue contained infiltrating ductal carcinoma *in situ* (cancer cells that infiltrated the duct but remained "in position," localized, inside the duct) and that clear margins had not been achieved when the tumor was removed. In addition, a second lump of approximately two centimeters existed within a different location of the same breast.

I sought opinions from two female and two male surgeons in three states. All recommended either a partial or a full mastectomy, lymph-node dissection, and follow-up therapy of radiation if the lymph nodes were negative or chemotherapy if the nodes were positive.

Ten days after my diagnosis, but before making any decision about further surgery, I began an intense immune system–building program that included a macrobiotic diet, affirmations, visualizations, yoga, meditation, psychotherapy, acupuncture, and Oriental herb remedies.

One month later, I concluded that no surgeon was willing to perform the type of surgery I wanted—a nondeforming procedure to remove only the remaining cancer tissue. I decided against chemotherapy, since that could impair my ability to have children and weaken my immune system. Radiation was not an option for me because I was extremely sensitive even to x-ray–level radiation (which is significantly less than the level of radiation therapy). I decided to stay with my self-designed program for two more months, hoping to preserve my breast as well as my ability to have children.

After only six weeks, miraculous changes began to occur: my chronic asthma, eczema, and sinus problems disappeared, as did my general fatigue, low energy, and gloomy outlook. I became confident that the program was working. After five months, the two-centimeter lump suddenly dissolved overnight. Six months later, I began to regain all the weight I had lost during the early stages of my diet change. One year later, when my annual mammogram was taken, the radiologist confirmed what I had suspected for six months: there was no more cancer. Nonetheless, after I had spent two years eating a careful diet, using herbal remedies, and practicing a variety of alternative treatments, my cancer came back in the same location as the original biopsy. I now had a five-centimeter tumor. I suspected that this time my lymph nodes were also involved, and therefore I decided to have a bilateral mastectomy in April of 1991.

If I knew on the day I was asked to return for a "simple little biopsy" what I know today, most likely I would have done things differently. I would certainly have interviewed surgeons and explored the possible outcomes *before* I had the biopsy. Instead, I forfeited my first choice by allowing the nurse practitioner—whom I had consulted about the lump—to schedule an appointment for me with the "first available" surgeon.

After my biopsy, I would have continued to search for a surgeon who would support my rights (1) to understand the treatment limitations and (2) to participate in my treatment decisions. I didn't lack access to the best medical treatment; rather, I lacked the self-confidence to insist on knowing my rights as a potential cancer patient. I lacked the background and experience to know that the lumpectomy and no radiation treatment I initially requested was both sensible and realistic given what the surgeons knew about *in situ* breast cancer.

When a second one-centimeter tumor was detected in my other breast, I once again declined having either chemotherapy or radiation (for reasons that I explain in detail in this book) and opted for alternative therapies. In July 1992, I had another recurrence, on the mastectomy scar near the original biopsy site. This half-centimeter tumor was also removed surgically. Once again I considered chemotherapy and radiation, but again declined this treatment. After an extremely stressful winter, I experienced still another recurrence. This time I had multiple tumors in my lymph nodes surrounding the site of the original tumor. After a short-lived attempt to use tamoxifen, I had an oophorotomy at the recommendation of my oncologist in May of 1993. Five weeks later the tumors vanished. Presently my cancer is in remission.

Patients have traditionally had very little to say about how their breast cancer is treated. I suffered from the rejection and abandonment often afforded to "noncompliant" patients, and therefore I started looking elsewhere for information and answers. My path back to health was not direct. I had to discover for myself what my treatment options and rights were. I wanted to know what had caused my breast cancer because I wanted to make certain that how I was living or what I was being exposed to would not be counterproductive to my efforts to recover.

The world of medicine has long perpetuated an attitude of "collective denial" by promoting the belief that breast cancer is curable if discovered at an early stage. Breast cancer is in fact a chronic disease, and at this moment it is not truly curable. "Curable," when used to describe breast cancer, refers to five-year survival rates. Recurrences are all too common. The drugs being used aren't "standardized" and therefore keep changing. Treatment options involve mutilation, radiation, and poisoning of our bodies. Breast conservation unfortunately doesn't provide any better survival than the out-dated Halsted radical mastectomy, albeit initially it gives women the opportunity to remain whole a little longer. And even after a woman has endured horrible treatments, no one can truly give her a clean bill of health.

Women with breast cancer are often led to believe that if they remain "cheery and hopeful" this too is helpful to their treatment and well-being. As long as women are given false reassurances about their breast-cancer diagnosis, we run the risk of becoming not only victims of the disease but also victims of the medical treatment itself. When people are victimized, they often feel too weak to fight back and too scared to question authority. This victimization serves to perpetuate outdated belief systems, in terms of both health care delivery and restorative medical procedures.

Long ago, patients victimized by cancer stopped questioning the out-of-control epidemic that is plaguing our nation and bankrupting our health-care system. Billions of dollars spent on research have not produced any definitive answers about how to prevent cancer or how to cure it. Cancer patients perhaps are too afraid to speak against the medical profession because, like battered women, they are dependent on the very persons who are responsible for the victimizing situation. While physicians may have the very best intentions, they, like batterers, are reluctant to see their own role in this debilitating scenario.

It seems to me that one of the reasons people who get cancer—any type of cancer—often feel like victims is that cancer has remained *mysterious.* When something is mysterious we can't help but feel helpless. Cancer seems to come from out of the blue and steal lives.

I have a medical-doctor friend who compares this "hard luck" attitude people have about getting cancer to that of some silly happenstance—like having a bird poop on your head. "Everyone," he says, "seems willing to accept cancer, like it was an accident or something." And so most people feel completely resigned when diagnosed.

In the afterword to *The Healing Heart,* by Norman Cousins, Dr. David Cannon describes how patients are "willing to put themselves completely in the hands of their physicians and exist in something akin to a state of suspended animation." Although he is writing about the heart patient, this same disconnection applies to patients with cancer as well. Needing to search for information after a devastating diagnosis seems like a huge obstacle. Knowing where to start, and taking the time and energy to do an exhaustive search before making life-changing medical decisions, can be overwhelming. The diagnosis alone causes some women to shut down just to protect themselves. But breaking out of the role of victim requires that we speak up for what we want for ourselves and for future generations.

The unspoken treatment premises are that a few more years of life at whatever cost is enough, that it's okay to exchange wholeness for life, that it's satisfactory to explain the source of breast cancer as multicausal or unknown. These are the rationales that are driving the approach to breast-cancer treatment today. Breast cancer is "managed" by the medical establishment with little presumption or even hope that it can be prevented.

Physicians themselves must nevertheless approach each woman's breast cancer as a fresh opportunity to beat the odds, and they, like their patients, have been conditioned to cope optimistically with the dismal history. Otherwise, how could they continue to practice, seeing the majority of their patients succumb to the disease? "A breakthrough in cancer treatment is just around the corner" has been the message in one form or another for decades, while many physicians and researchers continue to act as though it's not necessary to know the cause of breast cancer to treat it effectively.

There is no conspiracy in the medical system. Many doctors and research scientists have published papers and made public presentations echoing that no one is happy about the escalating incidence of breast cancer. No one is satisfied that one-fourth of all women who are diagnosed with the disease will die as a result of it within the first five years. No one likes having no alternative to performing ineffective treatments. Still medical practitioners seem to be educated to promote optimism. Medical researchers study and restudy the same old treatments—

believing that they are getting closer because another combination, duration, strength, or other variable will make all the difference.

I believe that the answers to how one gets cancer and how it spreads may already exist, but that it is difficult to see the cause of some cancers because they are evident only in a fragmented form. Like a jigsaw puzzle that has not been put together, the picture is impossible to make out because the assemblers are looking only at the few puzzle pieces directly in front of them. Currently no single research group is working strictly to assemble all the pieces of this puzzle. Instead, everyone is competing for limited research dollars to examine their particular viewpoints a little more closely.

Without bringing all the pieces together, how would researchers be able to identify what is missing? Could it be that the answer has been discovered over and over again but that no one can see it?

Believing in this possibility, I started my quest by asking: What is known about cancer? Where does cancer come from? How is cancer defined? These questions must occur to every person who gets this disease; I was no different. One of the most thought-provoking things I learned was that breast cancer doesn't have just one cause; it has many causes. What I didn't understand when I first heard this, from an epidemiologist at the National Institutes of Health (NIH), is that it applies to women both individually and collectively. Not only could my breast cancer have had more than one cause, but my premenopausal breast cancer and the breast cancer of a woman in the same town who is eighty-five years old are most likely caused by different factors. Women living in Japan may be given still different explanations for their breast cancers.

I also learned that some facts have long been known about cancer:

- Cancer is caused by something that is not natural to the human system.
- Cancer is the uncontrolled growth of cells.
- Cancer cells are not automatically detected by the body's natural immune system.

So "cancer," the uncontrolled division of cells, is caused by a genetic disposition or a mutagenic substance *outside* the body, substances we now know as "carcinogens." These foreign, toxic substances enter our system and interfere with our natural cell-producing functions as well as with our inherent ability to remove these abnormal cells.

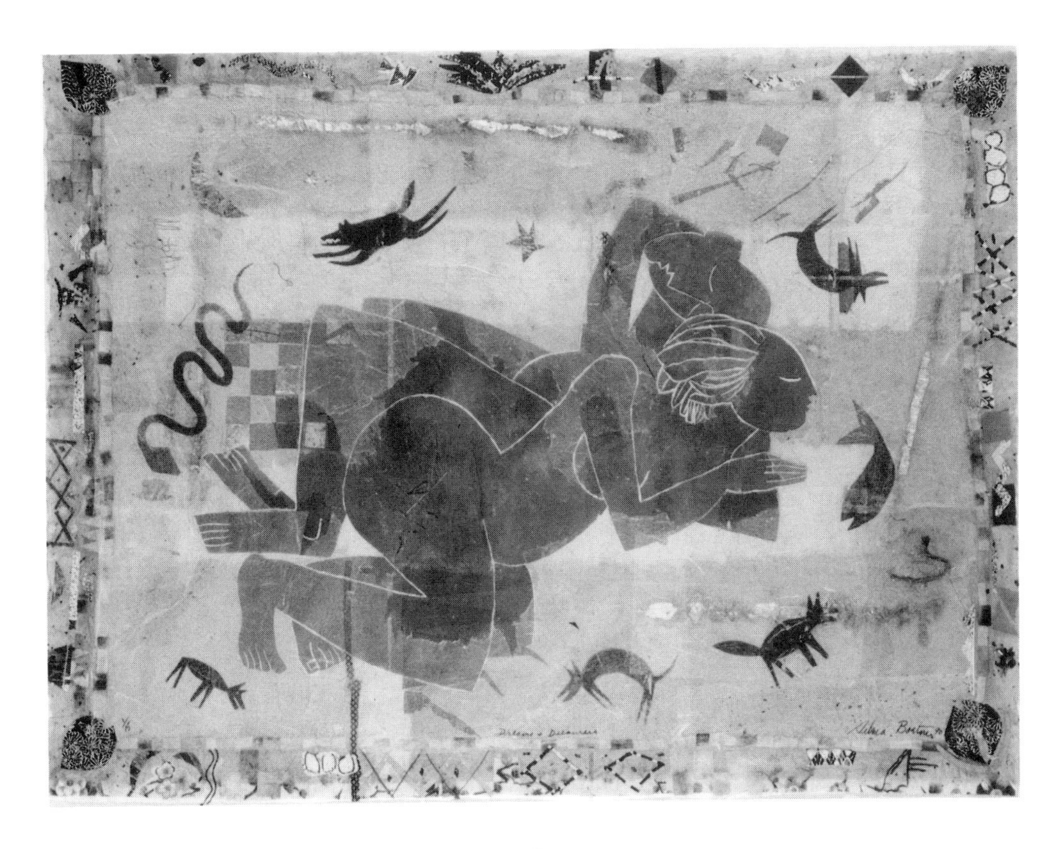

Dreams & Dreamers
Selma R. Bortner, Levittown, Pennsylvania
Collograph and collaged print with drawing, 28" x 32", 1989

"I was sixty years old at the time of surgery. I recuperated, taking sick leave for the spring semester, and went back to work full time in the fall of 1987. Retired in 1990, to get on with my own artistic development."

Breast cancer is a lesson for humankind. Our bodies are saying, "Hey folks, you are screwing up. It's time to stop and take a long, hard look at what you're doing in this life." We need to look at the environment, what we put in our bodies, and what we think about. This is our collective opportunity. Every woman diagnosed with breast cancer can make a difference in her own life. We can no longer demand fat studies while we continue to eat a high-fat animal-based diet, or express concern about the environment without making an effort to find a substitute for using balloons at our rallies and Styrofoam cups at our meetings. Becoming informed carries with it a responsibility to make both personal and planetary changes.

Initially my fight was a personal one. I was fighting for my life and I was fighting to stay whole. Now I'm fighting for more knowledge by exposing the dreadful lack of information that underlies breast-cancer treatment. Novel research projects and adequate funding have been absent because of the lack of patient constituencies willing to put themselves on the line by speaking up for better treatment, for a better understanding of the causes of breast cancer, and for prevention. This old model is finally being challenged.

It is no longer reasonable to resign ourselves to a disease that, no matter what its causes, has a destructive path. AIDS patients cope directly with knowing the truth about their illness: There is as yet no cure. The drugs and other treatments prescribed are experimental. The same is true for people with breast cancer. Like AIDS patients, we have to do whatever we can to fight our disease and to stay alive. And the causes of our disease must be identified, publicized, and prevented wherever possible. We, along with our doctors, need to face the facts of breast cancer and move forward as equal partners.

In *The Journey Beyond Breast Cancer* I explain how I approached my diagnosis so that others can see that there are options. This information is not necessarily provided so other women will follow my path, but because I believe women with breast cancer deserve to be told the truth about their illness. I believe we need to get beyond our denial to recognizing the seriousness of this epidemic and the role we have in changing its course on both a personal and a societal level.

PART ONE:

Searching for Courage

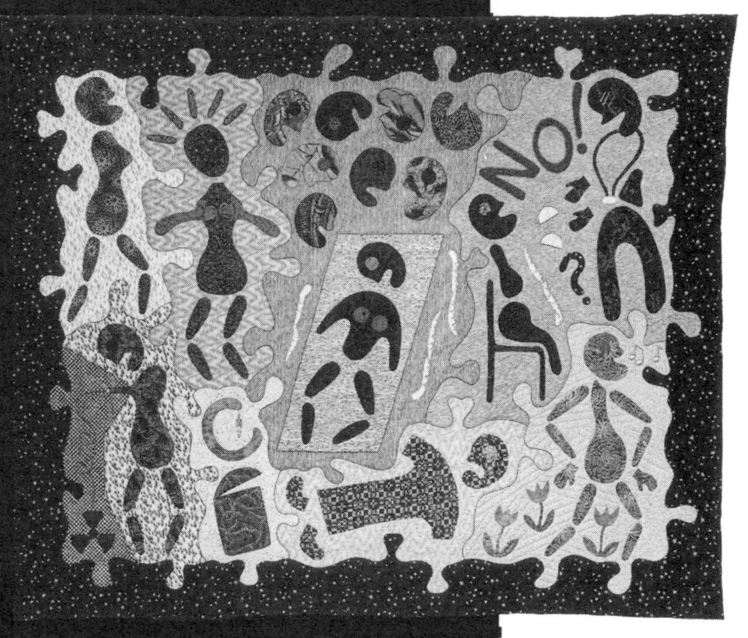

The Mastectomy by Suzanne Marshall

"The Mastectomy quilt was made for several reasons: First, I wanted to attempt making a non-traditional quilt and decided to try something in narrative form. Second, since my bilateral mastectomy nearly four years ago, I have been alarmed when hearing stories about women who have found lumps but have not sought treatment because of an overwhelming fear of disfigurement. I hoped to portray a positive message in a quilt—a changed body isn't what is important—LIFE IS! Third, I hoped to make a quilt that would stimulate conversation about a topic not discussed very much. Maybe if women would talk about breast cancer, it might not be as scary. And fourth, I have a concern that many women do not realize that they have a real choice regarding implants or cosmetic surgery. It is not necessary to conform to society's image.

The quilt is stitched in a puzzle form—after all, a diagnosis of breast cancer is something of a puzzle to be faced and needs to be taken one step at a time."

The Mastectomy
Suzanne Marshall, Clayton, Missouri
Fabric appliqué and quilting, 52" x 65", 1992

1

Finding My Own Way

The human body is its own best apothecary . . . because the most successful prescriptions are those filled by the body itself.

Norman Cousins

It takes courage for a woman to listen to her own goodness and act on it. For thirty-eight years, at the first sign of an ache or pain, the doctor was the first person I called. I have relied on doctors and what they are capable of doing all my life, and I still have enormous respect for the medical profession. Why then did I decide to reject the medical recommendations offered soon after I was diagnosed as having Stage I breast cancer?

Like the child who grows up and moves away from the shelter of her parents, I had reached the time when I needed to take charge of my own life. This didn't mean I no longer valued or asked for a doctor's opinion or help. But doctors, too, have limitations on what they know, and I decided that to face cancer I needed to develop my own values and measures for success.

For me, cancer represented a lesson in finding my own way. I was unwilling to turn my destiny over to someone else by entering the standard cancer-treatment program, which to me was the same as relinquishing every aspect of my soul and my body to a virtual stranger. I know my body and my health history better than any other person. I decided to seek out expert opinions and then to make the best decisions I could based on what I knew about myself.

When doctors are called upon to make decisions for their patients, they may make assumptions without comprehending personal details that would otherwise influence the decision. Part of my own decision-making process, for example, was rooted in having watched my mother die of colon cancer, from having seen a colleague's success in fighting breast cancer, and—perhaps especially—from my experience as a cross-eyed child.

My condition, strabismus, made it a struggle for me to learn to read; trying to make out what I was looking at was often confusing and resulted in frequent headaches. This experience taught me at an early age what it is like to be different physically. I soon learned how to compensate for my visual inadequacies: I avoided reading aloud in class, and I also avoided looking at another person straight on, in order to deter observation of my less-than-perfect appearance.

I was five years old when my mother began taking me to specialists—dozens of them over the years—but the doctors all said that my condition was not serious enough to risk the surgery required for a cosmetic correction. They couldn't explain why my eyes crossed, but they all seemed to concur that it wasn't a muscle problem but rather resulted from a lack of coordination between my eyes and my brain.

I lived with the stigma and handicap of being cross-eyed until I was thirty-seven years old, and then I learned of a surgeon who had perfected a technique that could straighten my eyes. Although I still have monocular vision, I am no longer cross-eyed. And it wasn't until I began my cancer research that I uncovered medical records from my infancy and a possible explanation for how I lost my eye-brain coordination: through the early administration of phenobarbital prescribed for colic.

The impact of these events and my personal history with specialists played a large part in my decisions about cancer treatment. For instance, I felt that just because a procedure was unknown or not currently in practice didn't mean it would always remain unavailable to me. Granted, breast cancer is life-threatening and strabismus isn't. Nonetheless, the medical treatments offered would only buy me time, and therefore I had to evaluate them: What were the known long-term carcinogenic ramifications of the standard treatments? How did they compare with the lesser-researched consequences of therapies that might also buy me time and be less likely to cause new cancers? What were the procedures *I* needed to heal?

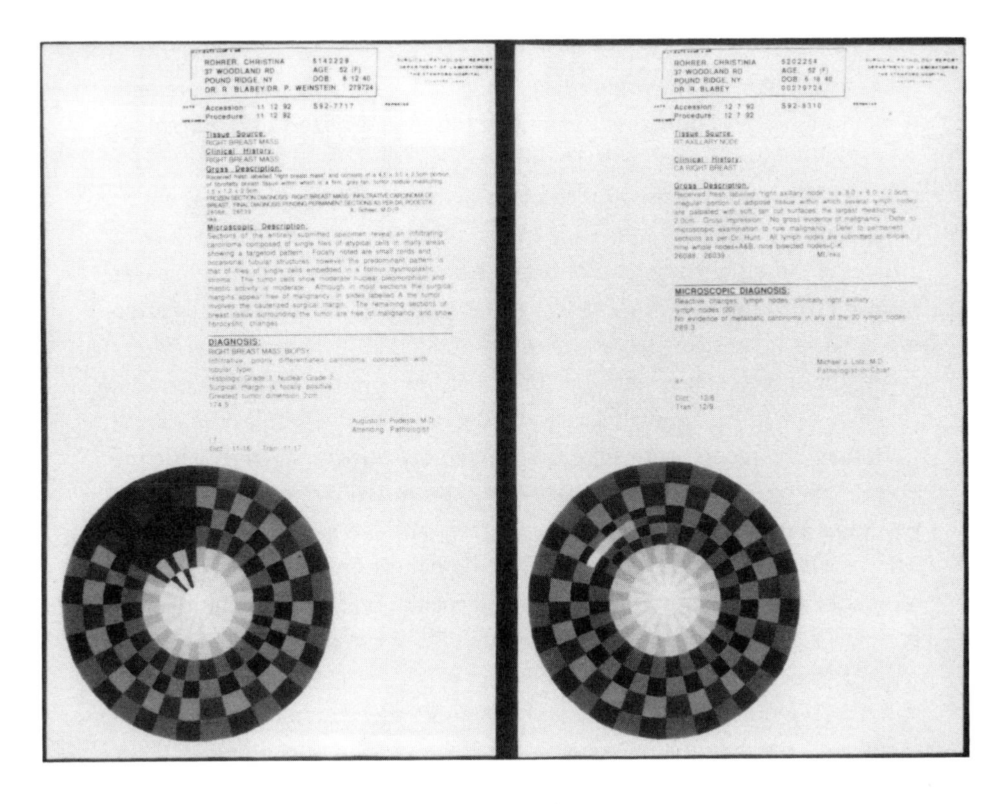

Hurting/Healing

Tina M. Rohrer, Pound Ridge, New York

Acrylic, xerox on paper, 18" x 24", 1993

"My initial reaction to my diagnosis was fear and anger. I wanted to cut out sections from certain wood constructions I had previously made. The appropriate tool would have been a chain saw. . . . The typographical errors in the medical reports . . . somehow reinforced my feelings of violation. Was I an error, too? Again reason prevailed and I realized that cancer was not a punishment for past mistakes. On the contrary, some of the nicest people I know are afflicted with this dreaded disease. It just happens."

MY GOALS

As soon as I learned that my breast cancer was probably eight years old, even though it was only one centimeter in size, I realized I wasn't going to die tomorrow or next year. The urgency to "do something" was also part of a learned response and fear that says "the sooner you get it out the better." Even this isn't certain, I learned; although some cancers are faster growing than others, my type of breast cancer was the slow growing kind. I was going to fight for more than the five years the doctors were predicting. I made a decision to take the time I needed to learn everything I could about my disease and how to stop it. I was in the fortunate position to make saving my life without sacrificing my dignity my full-time job.

Initially my goals were simple. I wanted the physicians to provide the nondeforming, lifesaving treatment that is promised by public health programs to women who get mammograms and whose cancer is detected early. I questioned the conventional treatment for breast cancer—surgery, radiation, and chemotherapy—and the expectation that women unlucky enough to contract cancer should put up with whatever treatment is recommended. I was unwilling to accept what was really unacceptable, and I rejected the "no pain, no gain" attitude we have been conditioned to accept—the idea that we must suffer in order to be successful in removing cancer.

Like most women in this situation I wanted to stay whole. I wanted to save my breasts *and* save my life. For me it wasn't an either/or situation. As women we are socialized to feel that our breasts are basic to our identity. When we face this life-threatening disease, the messages become more complex, depending on who we listen to. Doctors, family members, and friends can suggest everything from "You should simply live without them" to opposing or denying removal of the noninvolved breast simply because it is not required. It isn't uncommon for a woman facing a mastectomy to consider, a least for a minute or two, having her second breast removed for balance and added peace of mind, or to avoid a second surgery at a later date. Unfortunately, some doctors oppose this kind of request and will refuse to do such surgery. At the other extreme are women who are fighting to preserve their breasts at all costs. I could see there were no easy answers.

I envisioned the ideal treatment as being able to repair my whole system so I could be healthier, not weaker. I was convinced that my body had the internal capacity to eliminate the cancer itself if I could find a way to restore my natural immunity. What I wanted were techniques to:

- analyze the status of my lymph nodes without removing them,
- determine with precision the amount of tissue that needed to be removed, so that minimum mutilation would achieve the desired results, and
- provide treatments that wouldn't cause deformity or debilitate my immune system.

Then I asked, Can the doctors offer me this? The answer was no. These procedures aren't available. I sought out the best doctors in Vermont, Massachusetts, and Connecticut, looking for another way. After I made every attempt to find someone who would work with me in a personalized way to help me regain my health, I realized with disillusionment that I had no choice but to take responsibility for my own treatment and life. The procedures I would have preferred are outside the realm of the pathology techniques, surgery, and systemic treatments available in traditional hospitals today.

I suspected this might be different someday. I was aware of the impact Bernie Siegel and Norman Cousins were having on the old attitudes of the medical system. But meanwhile, I decided, I probably needed my lymph nodes more than they needed to be analyzed. Removing lymph nodes has little to do with preventing the spread of breast cancer; they are removed to determine the stage of the cancer. I wanted my lymph nodes (the filtering system of the body) to help me eliminate the cancer cells. This seemed to be a far more vital function than staging or assigning a protocol to my case.

SEARCHING FOR A PATH

Since I chose not to follow the standard procedure, I had to find an alternative route. This was very scary for me. I was in new territory and my life was at stake. I knew nothing about Oriental medicine, macrobiotic eating, homeopathy, or any other so-called New Age treatment.

This sort of personal crossroads is perhaps a point where some people become stuck. At the point of reckoning where we as newly diagnosed cancer patients need to choose a direction, one option is suddenly and irrevocably withdrawn: we cannot just go on as before. No matter what we do, *something* will change. I realized it was up to me to choose how much I wanted to participate in these changes.

When I first heard that I had breast cancer, I wanted to do anything but take responsibility. Fear of death took over my otherwise rational and educated mind, and the road of least resistance seemed to be to allow someone else to take charge. As I was considering the options offered, I felt a wide range of emotions. Bargaining became my dominant reaction. Yet, one thing I didn't want to bargain with was the idea of giving up a part of my body, my identity. Trying to absorb this new reality, I sometimes shut down my feelings, plunging into work and household activities and acting as though nothing would be different.

I wanted to find some way to get over my fear of cancer and learn to live more deliberately after the diagnosis. I didn't want to make my decisions from a position of utter terror. I kept saying I wanted to make my decisions with both eyes wide open, but I also realized this was going to be the hardest thing I would ever do.

I turned to God to help me through this initial fear and to bring into my life the kind of people who knew about alternative methods of healing. My business associate's approach to fighting her metastatic breast cancer contributed a great deal to my decision to try diet, meditation, and psychotherapy as my first line of defense. Reading in Fritjof Capra's *The Tao of Physics,*[1] a book about martial arts and practicing meditation, helped me to set my goals and to formulate my own plan of action. In the Buddhist tradition, being a warrior doesn't mean fighting; rather, it has to do with courage, strength, and patience—being prepared in every way so that the fight becomes unnecessary.

I wanted to participate in the choices to be made. I recognized that a doctor's words would, as always, carry enormous weight with me, so I asked my doctors to share with me both their knowledge and their limitations. This was a whole new world of language and information for me. To participate in my own treatment, I wanted to stay mindful and alert to new possibilities and approaches as well. Gradually denial became less of an issue. I evaluated each treatment individually based on what I felt was most suitable for me, weighing the best advice I could get. But as I looked for doctors who would respect my goals and treat me as a human being capable of making these decisions, often I didn't feel my questions were being answered with the thoroughness they deserved. I knew very little about this subject, and yet my doctors acted as though I was taking up too much of their time.

Since then, I have heard so many other women describe having had this same experience that I think many doctors really don't want to be challenged. They are tired of explaining the grim probabilities, and they hope for blind compliance. When I verbalized my understanding of the significance of my disease—that my life was in danger—and my desire for my illness to be treated with the seriousness it warranted, I found it more difficult to find supportive physicians.

Therapy helped me learn to ask people not to treat me as if I were dying—or worse yet, already dead (as I felt when people talked about me instead of *to* me). If anyone should have understood the importance of respecting a patient, it should have been the medical professionals. Unfortunately this wasn't my experience. It seemed as though neither the doctors nor my friends had confronted their own mortality. Instead of understanding, I got a wide range of reactions: distancing, ignoring the subject or me, downplaying the seriousness of my decisions, feeling sorry for me, coerciveness, and misinformation. What I needed was compassion, time, caring, information, understanding, respect, hugs, and love.

Even after I decided to follow my own path, I was terrified that at some point my doctors would desert me. Fear can be a powerful deterrent. As long as I felt fearful, I tended to be helpless and compliant. Knowledge became my response to this fear. Whenever a physician fostered fear in me, I considered that perhaps he or she was trying to manipulate me into being compliant and even dependent. It also occurred to me that this could be a signal to change physicians. I felt outraged that a doctor might want to exert this kind of power over me, over my life and my decisions.

Treatments for breast cancer today seem to be dictated more by the disease than by regard for the personal, emotional, and physical resources and needs of the patient. Women are instructed in what to do without really being given the opportunity to make choices. Our options are determined by a randomized combination of staging, chemotherapeutic protocols available in our region, and interpretation by the physician. Doctors are placed in the god-like role of deciding what is best for women even when there are no definitive results. Control is taken away from the patient until the doctors run out of treatment options. Then the

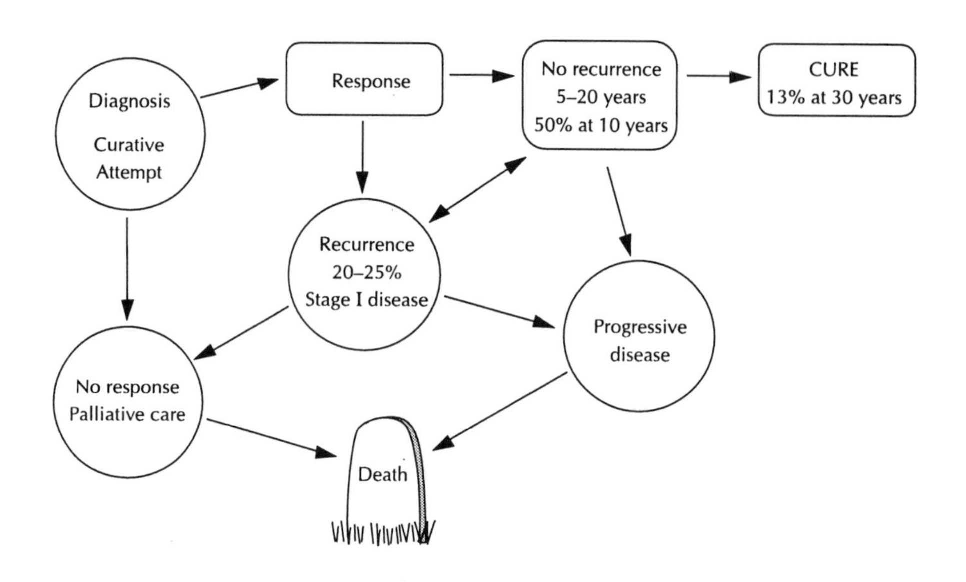

FIGURE 1
THE MECHANISM AND EVOLUTION OF BREAST CANCER TREATMENT

doctor delivers the hopeless pronouncement, "There is nothing else we can do," and the responsibility suddenly reverts back to the patient.

From this point on, pain management is all the doctors can offer. The patient has no immune system left and little strength to negotiate new options. Being aware of this evolution I decided that my best hope was to explore all my options while I was still strong, not waiting until I had run out of more traditional possibilities.

On the other hand, some people with cancer conclude that if they "do everything"—diet, herbs, meditation, chemotherapy, radiation, surgery—maybe something will pay off. But treating cancer in this shotgun fashion is not a strategy at all, because some treatments may work in opposition to one another. For instance, several of my friends attempted to combine a macrobiotic diet with chemotherapy. This proved to be especially difficult, since with chemotherapy their weight began to drop and they constantly craved fatty foods. Finally they decided that having the body weight was more important than eating healthy foods.

I believed that if a weakened immune system was the key to deterioration of health and the birth of a cancerous tumor, it was not in my best interest to subject myself to treatments that would weaken my already battered system. I was willing to see if I could get the upper hand on my cancer by ridding my body of toxins and restoring my immune system. I figured my odds were as good as the ones the doctor was giving me. How could I feel that I had failed if my cancer returned when I knew that 50 percent of the women diagnosed have recurrences in ten years? I wasn't living under the illusion that breast cancer was curable. I accepted it is a chronic disease.

I wanted a normal life expectancy. Perhaps this was fantasy or denial, but I was ready to fight to live until I was ninety. The more I researched my situation, the more I realized there were no simple formulas to follow. The doctors didn't have all the answers and neither did the alternative practitioners. If I wanted to be an enlightened consumer, I would have to dig up the information I needed, weigh my options, and take responsibility for my own decisions.

2

Searching for the Cause

Illness, physical or mental, could be a result of many things—not just what went into the human stomach, but also what went into the mind: relationships with family, friends, and the outside world; ambitions, hopes and fears.

"Jolly" West, M.D.

When I heard I had breast cancer, the first thing I wanted to know was *Why?* What caused it? What could I have done differently to prevent it? After only one trip to the medical library, I realized that there was no shortage of research on breast cancer. But although cancer has been studied and restudied for 2,500 years, the sad truth is that no one knows about what causes breast cancer or how to prevent it. When I examined more closely the death figures for the past decade, I was shocked to learn that more Americans had died of breast cancer than all the men and women who had died in battle in the Persian Gulf, Vietnam, Korea, and both world wars combined.

HIGH-RISK GROUPS

The risk factors that have been identified and accepted by the medical establishment are hardly risk factors at all. A true risk factor should be translatable into prevention programs. Intervention programs have been successful for heart disease and lung cancer. In these situations, avoiding smoking, reducing cholesterol, and increased exercise can be promoted and reinforced as public health programs. Unfortunately, with breast cancer the single largest risk factor is being female.

The classic risk factors fall into two main categories: (1) personal—reproductive experience, menopausal status, disease history, and family history—and (2) environmental—diet, medication use, and exposure to environmental carcinogens.[1] The American Cancer Society and the National Cancer Institute more frequently talk about and research the first category—the personal.

TABLE 1

PERSONAL RISK FACTORS FOR BREAST CANCER

Risk Factor	Higher risk state
Socioeconomic status	Affluent
Race	Caucasian
Cyclic ovarian activity	More years of duration
Reproductive history	Nulliparity, late age at first birth
Benign breast disease	Atypical hyperplasia
Lactation*	No history of lactation
Parenchymal patterns	P2, DY pattern
Family history	First-degree relative
Cancer history	Previous breast, endometrial, or ovarian cancer

*Premenopausal cancer

Source: Curtis Mettlin, "Breast Cancer Risk Factors: Contributions to Planning Breast Cancer Control," *Cancer* Supplment 69, no. 7 (April 1, 1992), 1904–10.

TABLE 2

ENVIRONMENTAL RISK FACTORS FOR BREAST CANCER

Risk factor	Higher risk state
Exogenous estrogens	Prolonged use
Fat and calories*	Excessive consumption
Alcohol consumption	Daily consumption
Radiation exposure	High-dose exposure

*Postmenopausal cancer

Source: Curtis Mettlin, "Breast Cancer Risk Factors: Contributions to Planning Breast Cancer Control," *Cancer* Supplment 69, no. 7 (April 1, 1992), 1904–10.

TABLE 3

FACTORS LIMITING THE APPLICATION OF KNOWLEDGE OF RISK FACTORS TO BREAST CANCER PREVENTION

Absence of primary sources of risk
Long latency between intervention and effect
Nonmanipulable nature of risk factors
Absence of controlled trial evidence of effect

Source: Curtis Mettlin, "Breast Cancer Risk Factors: Contributions to Planning Breast Cancer Control," *Cancer* Supplment 69, no. 7 (April 1, 1992), 1904–10.

In *Dr. Susan Love's Breast Book,*[2] breast surgeon and oncologist Susan M. Love identifies separate categories for the hormonal and genetic factors placing women at risk for breast cancer (with percentages, when available, indicating attributable risk):

Personal:

- over age fifty-five
- personal or family history of breast cancer (25%)
- never had children
- number of full-term pregnancies
- first childbirth after age thirty (17%)[3]
- never breast fed[4]
- early menarche (younger than twelve) or late menopause (older than fifty-five)
- obesity (12%)
- height
- personal or family history of other cancers
- socioeconomic status and race: white, upper-class women are at higher risk

Environmental:

- hormone replacement therapy (8%)
- diethylstibestrol (DES) exposure
- using contraceptive hormones: the Pill, the morning-after pill
- exposure to ionizing radiation
- diet (26%), including consumption of alcohol or caffeine, maintaining a high-fat diet, or suffering from nutritional deficiencies
- geographic location: inhabitants of North America and Northern Europe are at highest risk

Other factors that contribute to risk are being examined more closely. Some of these include:

- virus
- electromagnetic radiation
- carcinogenic chemicals, pesticides, additives
- fibrocystic disease
- thyroid problems
- lack of exposure to sunlight
- stress or personality difficulties
- low level of exercise as an adolescent
- high-fat diet as a teenager

Love points out that 70 percent of women diagnosed have none of the "classical" (that is, personal) risk factors in their background. I clearly had one—I didn't have children. And although there is no history of breast cancer in my family, my mother died of colon cancer, which is considered by some to have a familial relationship to breast cancer.

Examining the external factors that put me at risk appeared more compelling. I had used oral contraceptives (suddenly the fact that these were hormones had much more meaning to me) from the age of nineteen, off and on, until I was diagnosed. I had a high-fat diet as a teenager and had difficulty digesting fats both as an infant and later as an adult. I did not take drugs or drink alcohol, but I did drink caffeinated sodas and one or two cups of coffee per day. I wasn't particularly athletic. My office was located very close to a high-power transmission-line tower; five days a week for the three years immediately before my cancer diagnosis, I was exposed to electromagnetic radiation under this electrical field. I was exposed to numerous environmental and occupational carcinogens. In art school I was exposed to rubber cement, resins, polymers, paints, and thinners. As an interior designer I was exposed to the out-gassing of carpet and fabric samples, furniture finishes, cleaning fluids, and gypsum board. I also had a history of thyroid problems.

My life had included various risk factors from infancy through the time of my diagnosis. Was any one factor more causal than the others? Dr. Love's statement that "breast cancer is what is known as a multifactorial disease"[5] seemed to ring true in my case. The relationship between dietary fat and cancer, and my own lifelong difficulty in digesting fatty foods—particularly dairy products—became my first area of investigation.

WHAT WE NEED TO KNOW ABOUT MILK

Breast-feeding vs. Formula

When I was born, in 1951, the popular opinion was that bottle-feeding babies was purer, safer, and easier. One paper from this time discusses "streamlining the infant feeding."[6] Judging by my pediatric records, it is unlikely that my mother ever tried to breast-feed me when I was an infant.

Simple formula-feeding gave mothers a new freedom. As a nutritional source, formula was popularly promoted as superior to mother's milk. Physical growth was observed to be more rapid on formula; the assumption in the medical community, therefore, was that it produced healthier babies.

What doctors didn't tell women in the 1950s about homemade formula was that the composition was not designed to be like a human mother's milk but rather to simulate the higher protein content of cow's milk.[7] Such formulas do not offer children the protective antibodies that mother's milk does, and whole cow's milk, which is now considered unsuitable for infants younger than six months, was given to infants like me at three months.

The homemade formulas of the 1950s consisted of evaporated or whole cow's milk, lactic acid, Karo corn syrup (dextri-maltose), and water. Homemade formula feedings were often supplemented with orange juice and cod-liver oil.[8]

The problem is that cow's milk differs from human milk in the proportion of fat, protein, and carbohydrates. Another problem is that babies who don't breast-feed never receive the benefits of colostrum, a special fluid secreted during the first two to three days after birth and before the onset of true lactation. Colostrum carries antibodies and lymphocytes as well as great quantities of proteins and calories.

Lactose Intolerance

Today, commercials and nutritionists tell children that milk "builds strong bones and bodies." Adults are told that the calcium-rich milk helps to prevent bone loss. What people don't often hear is that not everyone is able to digest milk[9] and, furthermore, that drinking milk can cause health problems such as high cholesterol, heart disease, osteoporosis, allergies, eczema and other skin problems, weakened thyroid function in adults, as well as diarrhea and colic in babies.[10, 11]

Manufacturers have begun to market products to make it possible for people to digest milk even if they are naturally lactose intolerant. People with lactose problems often claim that cheese and yogurt are more digestible, which is highly possible because these products are lower in lactose. (They are still high in fat and protein.) Dr. John McDougall, summarizing the available literature on consumption of dairy products, concludes that "continuous overstimulation of the immune system by dairy proteins may eventually lead to the breakdown of the immune system into this form of cancer [Hodgkin's disease]. Lactose intolerance is especially common among adult Blacks and Asians [eastern and Pacific], occurring in as many as 90 percent of these people." Other ethnic groups prone to lactose intolerance include Africans, Arabs, Jews, Indians, Pakistanis, Eskimos, and Native Americans.[12] I am of Middle Eastern descent, and studies show, without sufficient explanation, that breast cancer is more prevalent among American Jewish women.

I went back and reviewed the pediatrician's reports that my mother had kept in my baby book and noted that when I went in for my first checkup I was eleven days old. Already I had colic, abdominal distension, conjunctivitis, engorged breasts, and eczema.

It didn't seem too farfetched to wonder if there was some connection between the formula that I was allergic to as a child and my breast cancer. Why were my breasts engorged during my first few weeks of life? Our family doctor apparently did not make an association between my symptoms and the formula. Instead he prescribed "elixir of phenobarbital with every other feeding or every feeding if necessary."[13] Basically this solution served to "sedate" the symptoms of my lactose intolerance.

When I was a child, my allergies, skin problems, and gastrointestinal problems were all treated by specialists who knew how to address my symptoms but who never explored the causes. Throughout my life, no one ever identified my chronic sinus infections, asthma, eczema, dry skin, dry scalp, chronic eye infections, and sensitivity to pollens and dust as dairy intolerance. When I was diagnosed with breast cancer, however, I went off dairy products and was amazed to discover that all these lifelong problems soon vanished.

Dairy Products

Consumption of dairy products may hold risks related to breast cancer regardless of whether a woman is lactose intolerant. One such risk stems from the hormones fed to the cows to increase and extend their milk production. The hormones consumed by cows in their feed are later absorbed by anyone who consumes dairy products. (This passing on of ingested substances is evident in mother's milk as well; for example, if a woman has lasagna seasoned with garlic and a glass of wine for dinner while she is breast-feeding, the breast milk will taste and smell both garlicky and alcoholic.) Most dairy products are high in dietary fat and protein. Furthermore, breast tissue is composed of fatty tissue, which becomes a storehouse for substances the body is unable to utilize, such as PCBs and DDT.

FATTY FOODS, BODY FAT, AND ESTROGEN PRODUCTION

Because of my difficulty digesting dairy products and fatty foods in general, I had long ago given up french fries, potato chips, ice cream, and whole milk. They all caused me extreme abdominal distress and uncontrollable gas. Prior to my diagnosis, I ate a lean diet—fish at least two times a week, pasta regularly, and vegetables, which I even liked. As an adult I was not overweight and I exercised moderately, but as a teenager I ate a diet high in fat and was not particularly athletic.

Most people know that eating fatty foods can increase body fat and that exercise can decrease body fat. After I learned that there is also a relationship between dietary fat and estrogen production, and ultimately a relationship between estrogen levels and breast cancer, I wanted to learn more about the connections among all these factors. Since age of onset of menarche appears to be influenced by dietary fat, scientists are beginning to examine this developmental phase more closely.

Rose E. Frisch of the Harvard School of Public Health studied 5,400 college alumnae aged twenty-one to eighty.[14] She created two groups that were similar in terms of age, family history, smoking, age of menarche, and postmenopausal estrogen use and investigated the effect of the women's participation in sports on their risk of breast cancer and cancers of the reproductive system. She found that women who were not athletes in high school and college have twice the risk of such cancers. Women who exercise regularly at a young age may experience a delayed menarche and lower level of body fat.

Dr. Frisch also concluded that exercise influences the *type* of estrogen produced in the body, which may account for less proliferation of cells in the breast and reproductive tissues.

Dr. Susan Love also emphasizes that diet in adolescence may be a crucial factor in minimizing a young's woman's risk of getting breast cancer later. Speaking before the U.S. Senate Subcommittee on Aging in June 1991, on behalf of the Breast Cancer Coalition, she testified:

> What we are dealing with is a combination of a tumor and an immune system. Some tumors are very aggressive and will have spread before they are palpable. Some tumors are very slow growing and will not have spread even though they have reached a large size. . . . Breast tissue seems to be more sensitive to carcinogens during adolescence than it is after the first pregnancy. It may well be possible that the time to study a low-fat diet is at puberty rather than in postmenopausal women.[15]

"Vulnerability to breast cancer," writes Love, is in some way related to the "length of time between menarche and menopause."[16]

In countries with low-fat diets, young women don't begin to menstruate until age fifteen, sixteen, or even seventeen. In the United States one hundred years ago, it was more common for girls to begin to menstruate later as well.[17] Today, age twelve is considered normal. Early menses may indicate a corresponding rise in a young woman's estrogen level and an increase in the time period of her greatest vulnerability to breast cancer. This, along with late menopause and delayed pregnancy, has been implicated as one of the risk factors for breast cancer related to hormone production.

Dr. Robert Hoover of the National Cancer Institute summarized a recent presentation entitled "Strategies for Prevention of Breast Cancer" by observing, "The good news is that we know breast cancer is related to ovarian/hormonal activity. The bad news is that we have known this since 1896—almost one hundred years."[18]

As early as 1896 the *Lancet* documented the improvement in the survival of two breast-cancer patients who had their ovaries removed to suppress hormone production. The role of estrogen in causing breast cancer was first established experimentally by a French scientist in 1932: when estrone, a type of estrogen produced in the female ovary, was injected into male mice, three of the mice developed breast cancer. Follow-up studies supported this connection between estrogen and breast cancer in both male and female rodents. "The importance of this observation," says Dr. Sherwood Gorbach in *The Doctor's Anti-Breast Cancer Diet,* "is that estrogens can cause breast cancers in animals that, under natural circumstances, are at extremely low risk for developing this disease."[19]

In 1992, *Lancet* published a study that analyzed the records of 1,655 women born at Uppsala University Hospital in Sweden. The results suggested that women who weighed more than eight pounds at birth had a 30 percent greater risk of developing breast cancer, while women whose mothers experienced toxemia during pregnancy had a 75 percent decrease in risk. The results pointed to the mother's estrogen level during pregnancy as a determinant in her daughter's risk for developing breast cancer.[20]

"My work in the past was all about life, seeds and growth in a very positive way. It never occurred to me that anything growing could be other than good. Then in September 1991 I was diagnosed with breast cancer and that theory was pretty nicely blown to bits. Suddenly the word growth was synonymous with bad and dangerous."

Susan Bohm
Scarsdale, New York

Today scientists know that excess estrogen inhibits the transformation of lymphocytes into effective defenders against disease. Then why do *post*menopausal women develop breast cancer more frequently than premenopausal women? While we don't know the answer for certain, we do know that just because women stop menstruating doesn't mean they aren't producing estrogen. Estrogen is also produced in or released from the liver, adrenal glands, and fat tissue. Estrogen stored in fat cells is released when the ovaries cease to function, also releasing stored pesticides.

Estradiol and estrone, both of which are specific kinds of estrogen produced in the female ovary, have also been observed in the urine of pregnant women. This not only may indicate that pregnancy is a time of increased estrogen but also demonstrates that the female body has a mechanism for excess estrogen elimination. Although pregnancy interrupts a woman's menstrual cycle, it is still a time of increased estrogen.

THE PILL

A newspaper headline on December 1, 1989—"Statistics Verify Trend of More Women Giving Birth After Age Thirty"[21]—made me realize that my decision to delay childbirth wasn't unique. The Centers for Disease Control had reported, "More than a quarter million women thirty and older—250,304—gave birth for the first time in 1987, compared with just 56,728 in 1970." The Pill was my method of contraception, and when I started taking them in 1969, the pills were very strong. (The Food and Drug Administration had approved the Pill for healthy women in 1959, even though the safety had never been confirmed.) The contraindications my doctor discussed were primarily heart disease, blood clots, and smoking.

I took the Pill on and off for nineteen years. Whenever I wasn't in a relationship I would quit taking the Pill because I worried about side effects I was experiencing, including weight gain, leg cramps, moodiness, and breakthrough bleeding.

The most striking contrasts between being on and being off the Pill occured about a year and a half before my diagnosis. I had unusual stiffness in my limbs, dizzy spells, excessive thirst, slurred speech, an irregular heart rate, and restless sleep. My calves were extremely sensitive to any weight; even the bed sheets were too heavy. I had no energy and felt tired most of the time. When these symptoms developed, my doctor ordered a complete cardiological workup—electrocardiogram (EKG), Holter monitor, treadmill test, and magnetic resonance imaging (MRI)—to determine whether I had a heart problem or perhaps multiple sclerosis.

The conclusion was that my symptoms were a result of "stress." I asked my boyfriend to move out of my house and I gradually began to distance myself from him. I also stopped taking the Pill. To my surprise the symptoms did go away. I associated the improvement with my recognition that I had been in a stressful relationship.

After I had been off the Pill for about a year, I started having irregular periods, which was very unusual for me. I was also experiencing some new problems. Increasingly I became more food sensitive and had trouble digesting anything prepared with fat.

During my annual scheduled gynecological exam, I told my doctor about my irregular periods. He knew I had been a long-term Pill user; he also believed in the Pill and used it to treat menstrual problems. He suggested I go back on the Pill even though I did not require any contraceptive protection at the time. During my first month back on the Pill, I bled or spotted for the entire month. Because I moved across the country during the same month, I figured it was probably a stress reaction. Stress was a pat diagnosis that I had received from doctors for so many years I had begun to repeat it to myself. Soon my periods became regular again, and I forgot all about the problem. Three months later a lump appeared in my breast. I couldn't help but wonder if after years of excess estrogen, the Pill had pushed my system beyond those initial "mysterious and unexplainable symptoms" to breast cancer.

Kathryn Stuart Huffman took the Pill for only four months during 1968. Months later, around the same time I first began taking the Pill, Kathryn was diagnosed with breast cancer. She was only twenty-two years old. After her diagnosis and a radical mastectomy, she filed a malpractice suit against the pharmaceutical company that manufactured the drug because her doctors believed her vigorously growing cancer was related to the hormones in the Pill.

Kathryn, a young woman completing her doctorate in international law at Harvard University, never fully recovered after her mastectomy. Even though her health deteriorated rapidly, and the suit was settled outside of court and the files sealed, Kathryn was determined to warn other women of the dangers of the Pill. She died shortly after her courageous but painful deposition and court appearances were complete.

In "*First Do No Harm . . .*,"[22] her mother tells Kathryn Huffman's story and asserts that Pill packages began to carry warning inserts because of the suit filed by Kathryn. Yet even today, the inserts provided by the drug manufacturers seem to play down the relationship between breast cancer and oral contraceptive (OC) use. I have compared early inserts with currently used inserts to see how women have been warned of the potential dangers.

Here is an early version of the insert, provided circa 1976:

> Women who have or have had clotting disorders, cancer of the breast or sex organs, unexplained vaginal bleeding, a stroke, heart attack, angina pectoris, or who suspect they may be pregnant should not use oral contraceptives.
>
> Birth control pills are not recommended for women past the age of forty because they increase the risk of heart attacks. However, proper use of oral contraceptives requires that they be taken under your doctor's continuous supervision, because they can be associated with side effects which may be fatal. Fortunately, these occur very infrequently. . . . Although the estrogen in oral contraceptives causes breast cancer and other cancers in certain animals, it is not known whether or not oral contraceptives can cause cancer in humans. At this time there is not definite evidence that they do.[23]

A more recent version of the insert, dated May 1990, reads:

> The use of oral contraceptives is associated with increased risks of several serious conditions including myocardial infarction, thromboembolism, stroke, hepatic neoplasia, gallbladder disease, and hypertension, although the risk of serious morbidity or mortality is very small in healthy women without underlying risk factors. The risk of morbidity and mortality increases significantly in the presence of other underlying risk factors such as hypertension, hyperlipidemias, obesity and diabetes.[24]

Additionally, the package inserts claim that the use of oral contraceptives is not associated with an increase in the risk of developing breast cancer, and that a cause-and-effect relationship between oral contraceptive use and breast and cervical cancers has not been established.

On first glance it appears as though the studies that show a relationship are canceled out by the studies that disprove a correlation. As recently as April 1991, a report on the health effects of contraception by the nonprofit Alan Guttmacher Institute in New York stated, "Women who use birth control pills for many years have a lower lifetime cancer risk than women who never use the pill."[25] But a comprehensive review of the literature published in *Acta Oncologica* in 1989 by Swedish oncologist Hakan Olsson offers a different picture.

Olsson reviewed thirty-five case-control and cohort studies published in peer medical journals between 1977 and 1988. Of the animal studies included in the review, Olsson states, "All hormonal components of oral contraceptives have been found to be carcinogenic in animal models."[26] Studies before 1977 were not included in the review because these reports had defects in choosing the subjects for study or in establishing a consistent definition of contraceptive use.

Olsson reports that in studies comparing human OC users screened for breast cancer against screened controls who never used OCs, "fifteen out of seventeen [studies] reported an increased risk of breast cancer which could be correlated to the early use of oral contraceptives, even though investigation of this hypothesis was not the immediate aim of all studies."[27]

Out of these fifteen studies, eleven showed a "significant" increased risk. Two studies showed increase was affected by duration of usage. The two studies that had reported indications of reduced risk "were both based on the same material which, after the inclusion of more subjects and re-analysis by the same research group, showed a *significantly* [emphasis added] increased risk instead."[28]

Of the studies that occurred after 1985, six had defects such as the inclusion of insufficient numbers of young users, the inclusion of an age group that could not have used OCs at a very young age, or omission of the women's ages. Five studies remained, of which four demonstrated an increased risk. The one remaining study, from New Zealand, showed an increased risk for women twenty-five to thirty-four years of age after more than ten years of use; this statistic was not considered "significant."

In addition to a review of the published literature, Olsson examined statistics describing localities of high use of the early Pill, and he correlated this with areas of increased breast-cancer incidence. He reports, for example, that in the 1960s in Sweden, England, and certain regions of the United States—one being California—use of the Pill was more extensive among teenagers than among teenagers elsewhere.[29] Countries like France and Italy—which did not encourage extensive use of oral contraceptives by teenagers until ten years later than the United States and Sweden—currently have lower rates of breast cancer. It certainly would be worthwhile watching to see if their rates increase as these teenage users grow older.

Olsson furthermore explains that "it takes approximately thirty cell divisions before a malignant breast tumor can be diagnosed. . . .The latency time varies between ten to thirty years."[30] I was a teenager living in California during the late 1960s, so all these data were of particular relevance to me. I started taking the pill in 1969. My breast cancer was diagnosed in 1989. Essentially my generation—women who were in their late teens between 1967 and 1972—is the first generation that has used oral contraceptives long enough, and began early enough, to experience breast cancer as a consequence. Reading this review convinced me that taking birth control pills was a major factor in the ultimate development of my breast cancer.

In 1974, a woman with breast cancer named Rose Kushner began contacting the Food and Drug Administration, Congress, and the National Cancer Institute to find out why no one wanted to address the breast cancer/Pill connection. She was a one-woman activist movement until 1975, when a private attorney offered to take up the issue of legally requiring drug companies to provide more detailed patient warnings on the Pill package insert. After many hearings, a small victory was won in 1978: material previously contained in a separate patient booklet would be included on the insert. The required material, however, did not include any special warnings or restrictions for women with a family history of breast cancer.

Kushner believed that the issue of taking estrogen went beyond oral contraceptives, since she herself had never used the Pill but had begun taking hormones as a teenager. In *Alternatives: New Developments in the War on Breast Cancer,* she describes how the hormones had been prescribed over the years to regulate her menstrual periods, clear up her skin, prevent miscarriages, and dry up her milk.[31]

When traveling in Europe, Kushner found everyone she interviewed in agreement about the carcinogenic nature of oral contraceptives. "It seems everyone, everywhere, considers the Pill dangerous except women in the United States," she observes. But she emphasizes, "Whatever the seed might be, the estrogens in these drugs are fertilizers that stimulate and speed the growth of mammary carcinomas. Research literature shows evidence that, while OCs may not be carcino-*genic* in humans, they are certainly carcino-*trophic*—cancer-nourishing."[32]

Years of research later, however, even stronger evidence indicates that the Pill increases a woman's risk for breast cancer. A 1989 article entitled "Breast Cancer Before Age Forty-five and Oral Contraceptive Use: New Findings" in the *American Journal of Epidemiology* reported:

> This study provides new evidence to suggest that the risk of breast cancer is increased among women below the age of forty-five years who have used oral contraceptives. The risk appeared to be approximately doubled for use of less than ten years duration and quadrupled for ten or more years of use. The association was present in virtually all subgroups examined.[33]

The *British Journal of Cancer*[34] published an editorial in 1990 reviewing thirteen major case-control studies on the relationship of oral contraceptives to breast cancer in young women. Eight studies demonstrated that when the Pill is taken over an extended period of time (for more than eight years) and is started in a woman's late teens and early twenties, the risk of breast cancer increases. This evidence appeared applicable to early-age (before forty-five) breast cancer.

No one had this sort of information when the Pill was first offered. And it wasn't until I was diagnosed with breast cancer, and began to see more and more cases of breast cancer occurring in women under fifty, with no family history of breast cancer, and with children, that I started to take more seriously the conflicting studies about the safety of oral contraceptives.

OTHER SOURCES OF HORMONES AND DES

Joseph Highland and his co-authors cite in *Malignant Neglect,* "In 1977 the Occupational Safety and Health Administration fined a pharmaceutical house in Illinois more than $50,000 after male workers in DES production suffered from breast enlargement and impotency."[35] Some research studies suggest that the risk of breast cancer increases for the daughters of women who took diethylstilbestrol (DES) during the 1940s and 1950s to prevent miscarriage.[36] (It was later determined that not only was this drug dangerous, causing vaginal malignancies in the daughters of women who took it, but it was completely ineffective.)[37] Researchers from the National Cancer Institute testified to Congress that only one molecule of DES in a quarter pound of beef liver could trigger human cancer.

No amount of DES is considered safe. Nonetheless, the "morning-after pill," which contains 250 milligrams of DES, was made available in 1971 to healthy young women to abort fertilized ova, without FDA approval for this use. In 1973 it was approved by the FDA for "emergency" use. The 250 milligrams of DES in each pill is 55,000 times the amount the FDA tried to ban in cattle feed and 500 times the amount normally circulating in a woman's body.[38]

Our own ovaries, liver, and adrenal glands produce hormones, and hormone levels increase with a high-fat diet. That high-fat diet may consist of products from animals that also produce hormones naturally; in addition, most commercial livestock have been fed hormone stimulants to increase their body weight or milk production.

The FDA approved DES as a feed additive for cattle in 1954, as a means of producing more weight and fat on the animals. After concerns were raised about residues in meat for human consumption, the U.S. Department of Agriculture inspected meat samples in 1971. Residues were in fact found. In 1973, DES was banned, but a year later the ban was relaxed, and farmers were directed only to stop using DES in animal feed seven days before slaughter. In *Diet for a New America,* John Robbins reports that "farmers who accidentally absorbed, inhaled, or ingested even a minute amount of this drug . . . exhibited symptoms of impotence, infertility, gynecomastia (elevated and tender breasts)" along with other problems.[39] Several years after the ban went into effect, "no less than half a million cattle were found to have been illegally implanted with DES."[40] DES is only one of fifteen sex hormones that the FDA allows in animal feed, according to Robert Boyle and the Environmental Defense Fund.[41]

We don't know how the hormone residues that we ingest from commercially raised milk, meat, and chicken are utilized by our bodies or how they influence the way we store fat. The outcome depends on how much we consume, the duration of consumption, the type of hormones fed to these animals, and how they are stored in our fat tissue, liver, and colon.

Rose Kushner points out that attributing the cause of her breast cancer to estrogen use does not factor in the "gallons of chicken soup [DES impregnated until 1959] and the DES chopped liver [still DES contaminated] I had eaten in my life."[42] I too can't help but wonder about the countless numbers of women at risk for breast cancer—and how much of this substance we continue to injest in the animal products we consume.

MELATONIN AND HORMONAL HEALTH

Other factors controlling hormone regulation have been explored by cutting-edge scientists as diverse as research psychiatrists, energy scientists, and experts in endocrinology and metabolism.[43] Working independently, such researchers have examined connections between and among hormones, emotions, immune function, breast cancer, electromagnetic fields, and sunlight.

Much of this recent work focuses on melatonin, a hormone produced in the pineal gland—which helps to regulate the female reproductive cycle—that has been shown to inhibit the growth of breast-cancer cells. Melatonin, produced naturally by our bodies when we sleep, enhances the immune system and suppresses sex-hormones such as estrogen and testosterone.[44] When melatonin production is impaired, sex-hormone production increases and the immune system is weakened.[45]

So crucial is melatonin to other hormonal functions that a Dutch doctor named Michael Cohen in 1991 applied for a grant from the National Institutes of Health for further research of a new birth-control pill, B-Oval, that he claims will also prevent breast cancer, much as progestin helps ward off cancer of the uterus and ovaries. Cohen replaces estrogen, the main ingredient in most birth-control pills, with melatonin, which he has demonstrated inhibits the monthly flow of cells to the breast in preparation for lactation. Dr. Cohen theorizes that some cells may not disperse when the cycle progresses and a woman has not conceived. This "clumping," which is prevented by the use of melatonin, contributes to the creation of breast cancer.[46]

The *Los Angeles Times* reported in February 1980, "Rays of sunlight stimulate the pineal gland . . . [which] secretes melatonin, a hormone that . . . induces sleep, inhibits ovulation, and modifies the secretion of other hormones. Sunlight seems to be a significant influence in the regulation of melatonin."[47] And, indeed, after using "melatonin stimulation" with full-spectrum ultraviolet lights to create "indoor sunshine," scientists have observed that zoo and farm animals experience a boost in beef production (without increasing food consumption), increased egg laying, better milk production, greater fertility, and better adjustment to captivity.[48] In Russia, full-spectrum lights have been used for human beings to improve factory production, reduce absenteeism, improve student behavior, and reduce fatigue. Other positive effects of full-spectrum light in humans include control of jaundice in newborns, control of viral and cold infections, endocrine control, and enhanced immunologic responsiveness.[49]

Nonetheless, extremes of any sort can cause an imbalance in homeostasis. Excess melatonin may cause problems like chronic fatigue syndrome: the more a person sleeps, the more melatonin is secreted, which induces sleepiness—and a vicious circle results. (I can remember times when I didn't get out of bed at my normal time and thought, Oh, I'll sleep in this morning. When rising a few hours later, I felt groggy and more tired. Today I theorize this lethargic feeling may have resulted from excess melatonin, resulting from my body's attempt to balance a low estrogen level.)

The suppression of this powerful hormone has correspondingly negative effects, too. Energy researcher Richard Stevens maintains that melatonin is suppressed when we live near high-power transmission lines or are exposed to other energy sources with strong electromagnetic fields (EMF). According to Stevens, "This may explain why chronic EMF exposure is associated with increased rates of certain cancers."[50] As it happened, my office had been located next to a high-tension power line.

David Carpenter, a project researcher for the New York State Department of Health, estimated that 30 percent of all childhood cancers may be due to exposure to extremely low-frequency electromagnetic fields (LF-EMF), such as those produced by power lines.[51] The *Lancet* in December 1990 described the association between an "effect of light and LF-EMF on pineal melatonin production, and on the relation of melatonin to mammary carcinogenesis."[52] The journal stated the association between breast cancer and occupational exposure to ELF fields needs further study. A second study published in March 1991 suggests that the increased rates of breast cancer observed in male telephone workers may be connected to EMF exposure that changes melatonin rhythms.[53] Other scientists have specifically demonstrated a relationship between female breast cancer and exposure to overhead power-transmission lines near the home.

IONIZING RADIATION

Although the female breast is part of the reproductive system, it is still exposed to harmful radiation in the name of diagnostic procedures and treatment. Numerous studies demonstrate the overall, long-range effects of ionizing radiation (diagnostic and therapeutic x-rays). Studies of women who survived the atomic bombs dropped on Hiroshima and Nagasaki during World War II show that breast cancer increased most dramatically among women who had been in their teens and early twenties.[54] Women treated with fluoroscopy (daily chest x-rays) for tuberculosis during the 1930s and 1940s showed an increase in breast cancer, but those cancers have taken twenty to thirty years to develop.[55] Young girls exposed to multiple diagnostic x-rays for scoliosis have a nearly twofold risk of breast cancer. (These low-dose x-rays had an average cumulative breast dose of thirteen rads.)[56] Women who had high-dose radiation (fifty to four hundred and fifty rads) delivered to both breasts for treatment of postpartum mastitis (painfully inflamed breasts that occur during lactation) experienced higher rates of breast cancer,[57] as did women who as infants were haphazardly exposed to radiation treatments to the thymus gland because of its excess size. The thymus is located adjacent to the breast tissue, and the radiation treatment most likely included a larger area than the thymus itself.

To put doses of radiation in perspective, mammograms today average approximately two hundred and fifty millirads per breast for a two-view examination.[58] One thousand millirads equals one rad. In the 1970s, mammograms delivered six to fifteen rads per exam.[59] A chest x-ray today is about ten millirads per view. Therapeutic radiation to the breast is five to six thousand millirads. Both diagnostic and therapeutic radiation produce "scatter," which may accidentally affect the thymus gland, our storage center for cancer-fighting T-cells. T-cells are unique immune-responsive lymphocytes, which can survive for up to five years, indicating they do not reproduce at a fast pace.

For the first time, researchers are saying that x-rays to the breast may actually *cause* breast cancer. An article in the *New England Journal of Medicine* (December 26, 1991) reports that "Dr. Michael Swift and his colleagues at the University of North Carolina in Chapel Hill found the cancer link in people who carry the ataxia-telangiectasia (AT) gene. If someone inherits two copies of this gene—one from each parent" this disease shows up as affecting coordination. "However, about 1.4 percent of Americans carry one copy of the gene and suffer no obvious side effects." Swift's team showed that "nearly eight percent of all breast cancers in the U.S. could result from this gene [and that] radiation can trigger [the cancer].[60]

The disturbing thing about overall radiation exposure is that no one is keeping track. I couldn't say with certainty what my exposure for this past year has been, let alone my lifetime exposure. As it stands today, we are given fixed screening guidelines that do not take into consideration our individual circumstances. For example, radiation is shown to be greater than expected for those who fly often.[61] Should airline flight crews who have increased radiation exposure adhere to the same mammography guidelines as school teachers? Should a woman who has had therapeutic radiation treatment for scoliosis and is a frequent business flyer have annual mammograms?

When women express fears about the unknown long-term impact of mammograms, they are reassured by radiologists that mammograms are safe. Unfortunately, earlier assurances concerning radiation have later been determined to be false. One woman told me that when she went in for her routine mammogram, the first four views were taken without film and therefore had to be repeated. Then an additional two views were taken because the pictures were not clear. No guidelines currently exist for the number of mammograms that can safely be taken in one day or one year. Radiation usage, leakage, and testing have a history of careless and abusive practice, of which many people remain unaware. This leaves us all extremely vulnerable to both human and technological limitations and errors.

EMOTIONAL STRESS

A most disturbing discovery came when I read the pediatrician's instructions to my mother about picking me up or allowing me to be handled by my sister. The doctor wrote, "Joy and pleasure in the child should be gotten in giving the necessary service. Leave the infant alone. Much handling and indulgence, using the infant as a thing or object of amusement, will increase your present problems and will bring many emotional maladjustments."

Nothing could have been further from the truth about child rearing. Yet this trained physician told his patients, mothers like mine, that this was the best way to treat a baby. Exploring this advice with several psychotherapists raised my awareness that this was standard practice in the 1950s; perhaps it is one reason there are now so many insecure adults seeking self-help programs. It was the middle-class women who could afford to see a pediatrician regularly who were instructed in the latest techniques of child rearing: these children are the same children who now compose the largest population of women at risk for breast cancer.

As a baby I had to fend for myself. I was "serviced"—like a car, not a baby—because a doctor my mother trusted told her this was the way to raise a child. The odd thing was that my mother had already raised two daughters and breast-fed and handled both of them.

Because breast cancer is such a slow-growing cancer, the circumstances that will influence its development could in fact begin at birth and be altered by what transpires over the next twenty-five to thirty years. Emotional factors have been demonstrated to affect our well-being and immune systems. If we hope to someday prevent breast cancer or its recurrence, we are going to need to better understand what circumstances have broken down our immune system and then strive to remove these threats.

It's no wonder that scientists can confidently say that there are many causes of women's breast cancers. More accurately, breast cancer is perhaps "caused" by a long-term breakdown of the immune system that prevents it from eliminating dangerous cell mutations. Eventually our system becomes overwhelmed and a cancerous tumor develops. For this reason no one will be able to point a finger at any one culprit, like diet or the Pill.

The lack of this kind of conclusive information doesn't mean there isn't good reason to change our habits. For suggestions about how you can use what we know about possible causes, see the prevention list included in Part Three under "Choosing Life," and "Appendix 3: Reducing Your Breast-Cancer Risk Factors."

3

Deciding What To Do

Knowledge is the food of the soul.
Plato, 360 B.C.

Our ability to make intelligent decisions about our breast cancer treatment can be influenced by the amount of time we have to adjust to the diagnosis. A woman with breast cancer needs time to "mourn the loss of her health to a chronic disease with its ever-present threat of death and the loss of her intact body."[1] We may nonetheless find ourselves on a fast timetable as a result of our fears and the medical treatment schedules when facing the prospect of surgery, radiation, chemotherapy, and perhaps even breast amputation. These circumstances often prevent us from taking the time we need to fully "own" our decisions and their possible outcomes.

I wanted to know all the facts about my condition, the treatment options, and how my choices would affect my future. This was my life—the outcome couldn't be of greater concern to anyone else. I felt a need to analyze the medical treatments for breast cancer independently of what the doctor was telling me. I thought it was important to consider how the medical treatment itself might compromise my body's ability to recover from breast cancer, compared with how this disease might progress *without* treatment. So I turned to the medical library, examining periodicals, books, and data-base resources at the National Cancer Institute.

THE HISTORICAL RECORD

Beginning at the beginning, I wanted first to take a look back at how breast cancer has been treated historically. The Latin word cancer comes from the Greek *karkinos,* meaning "crab"; the fifth century B.C.E. physician Hippocrates, who had likened the long, distended veins radiating from lumps in the breast to crabs, used the Greek word *karkinoma.* All the discussions about the source and treatment of cancer in early medicine begin with *breast* cancer. This seems to be the condition attributable to the word *cancer* itself.[2]

L. J. Rather in *The Genesis of Cancer* quotes a Hippocratic writer describing *karkinoma* as "hard growths in the breast that do not suppurate but increasingly harden and develop into occult cancers. Pain extends from the breast region to the neck and shoulder blades and the body becomes wasted; treatment at this stage is without avail, and death ensues."[3]

Even though surgery was practiced by the ancient Greeks, Hippocrates considered "no treatment at all" superior to surgery, according to Michael Baum, a professor at King's College Hospital, London, who traces the history of early surgery in *Breast Cancer: The Facts.* Baum records that during the third century, mastectomy was used as a "punitive rather than a therapeutic weapon."[4] One eminent casualty of this punishment was the Christian saint Agatha. Having dedicated herself to God and a life of chasity, Saint Agatha rebuffed the advances of Quintian, a man of consular rank; in retribution she was subjected to numerous tortures, one of which was the amputation of her breasts.[5] In Greek and Roman art, Agatha is depicted holding a pair of pincers (used for breast removal) or bearing her breasts on a plate. (Over the centuries the breasts have sometimes been misinterpreted as loaves of bread.)[6]

During the Renaissance, several doctors recommended mastectomy as treatment for cancer of the breast. An early eighteenth-century physician named LaDran is credited with using lymph-node involvement for assessing prognosis (he described the outlook with lymph-node involvement as poor), and the French anatomist and surgeon Jean Louis Petit (1664–1741) advocated the "removal of the primary growth and the axillary nodes [lymph nodes under the armpit]."[7]

Although no data on survival rates were formally recorded, some women apparently did survive the surgical treatment for breast cancer. In

1700, Sister Barbier de l'Assomption was a nurse at what is now the oldest hospital in North America, L'Hotel Dieu in Quebec. The story is told that after discovering her breast tumor, she first put herself in the hands of God and then underwent an operation performed by the hospital's famous surgeon Michel Sarazan. Baum relates that she made an "uneventful recovery and did not die until thirty years later, by which time she had risen in the ranks to Mother Superior."[8]

By the middle of the nineteenth century, doctors had begun to keep records. The British surgeon Sir James Paget leaves behind a report typical of his time. Paget treated seventy-four cases of breast cancer with mastectomy and experienced a 100 percent recurrence rate within eight years. The gloomy picture is further elaborated upon by James Syme; writing in his textbook *Principles of Surgery* in 1842, Syme concedes: "It appears that the results of operations for carcinoma when the glands [meaning lymph nodes] are affected is almost always unsatisfactory, [no matter] how perfectly they may seem to have been taken away."[9]

In spite of these results, surgeons persisted in trying to "perfect" their procedures and continued to remove more and more tissue. In the 1890s, a widely accepted protocol was developed by the American surgeon William Stewart Halsted that called for removing the breast, chest-wall muscles, and neck and axillary lymph nodes. When that didn't work, physicians concluded that they needed to remove even more.

One reason Halsted's "radical mastectomy" became the popular treatment choice was that early publications claimed a high proportion of three-year "cures." These reports shed light on the origin of the misleading substitution of the word "cure" for survival.

Halsted and his students reported that nine hundred patients were operated on between 1889 and 1931, with the following results: 6 percent died soon after their operation, the local recurrence rate was 30 percent, and the ten-year survival rate was 12 percent.[10] This was a 3 percent improvement over the observations of Samuel Gross (1837–1889), an American surgeon who in 1880 published one of the first treatises on the treatment of tumors.

Gross described the status of breast-cancer treatment during the pre-Halsted era. Keeping in mind that most of the operations were carried out on advanced cancers, the following results are offered for comparison with Halsted's. Gross observed 660 cases, of which 70 percent had skin infiltration on presentation (the cancer in some way visible on the skin), 25 percent had skin ulceration. Two-thirds of the cases had "obviously involved axillary nodes," and a third had palpable supraclavicular nodes.[11]

Of the above 660 cases, 519 were treated by surgery: more than half by simple mastectomy, and the rest by mastectomies that included axillary-node removal. The results included 17 percent operative deaths, 80 percent recurrences, and 9 percent achieving ten-year survival. Patients with no node involvement typically survived more than six years. Postmortem studies proved that one in eight patients had secondary tumors in the bone, *without* glandular involvement. This finding led Gross to speculate that the "spread of the disease was via the bloodstream rather than the lymphatic system."[12]

Baum extols the work of Gross in 1880 as "truly remarkable observations which . . . have been rediscovered within the last thirty years, and form the basis of the contemporary biological model that describes the behavior of breast cancer."[13]

The staging of disease progression became popular in the 1940s in England with the Manchester staging system. This system described "Stages I and II representing the operable (curable) groups; Stage III the locally advanced disease where surgery was doomed to failure; and Stage IV the patient with obvious distant metastases." Baum attributes the improvement in ten-year survival from 10 percent in the 1920s to 50 percent in the 1950s to the "better selection" of patients for mastectomy resulting from staging.[14]

Although it has been observed that some untreated cancers can lead to an "inevitable and rapid death," breast cancer does not consistently follow this pattern. "Breast cancer," observes Baum, "can be a very slowly progressive disease, in spite of treatment, leading to the patient's death maybe twenty years after mastectomy. It is not surprising, therefore, that a number of women will die of other causes, even though not 'cured' of their original cancer" because the average age of onset is fifty-five years old. He goes on to point out that breast cancer "does not behave as a single entity but has an extraordinarily wide biological variation in behavior, with some women dying of the disease with an almost undetectable primary tumor, whereas others may live for many years after having refused treatment in the first place."[15]

Baum's statement is supported by his review of case studies from Gross's era to the present day. Furthermore, 10 percent of the untreated patients in Baum's review survived ten years without any treatment, a percentage equal to the survival rate of the women who underwent mastectomies during this same time period.

Dr. Bloom of the Royal Marsden Hospital in London studied the records of 250 women who died of breast cancer between 1805 and 1933. Some had undergone treatment, while others ignored the symptoms until they were in the final stages. Most of these patients had locally advanced or widely disseminated disease. An estimated 18 percent survived five years, and 3.6 percent for ten years *without* treatment.[16]

Baum cautions against using these studies as a "baseline against which to judge the curative effect of conventional therapy." These studies contained information about women seeking medical attention before "public health education had warned the population of the sinister significance of breast lumps. It is likely, therefore, that many women were content to co-exist with their breast lumps until they died of old age or were knocked down by a hansom cab."[17] Furthermore, self-selection—or withholding procedures from patients deemed to have a poor prognosis—distorted the results of early studies that sought to evaluate the curative effect of conventional therapy during the first half of the twentieth century.

In 1965 the Ontario Cancer Clinic offered the results of a statistical review supporting the idea that breast cancer has two types of behavior patterns: in one type, the cancer metastasizes early and "must be considered incurable by any form of local treatment"; a second type is nonmetastasizing—"or at worst does not start to metastasize until the lump has been obvious for a number of years"—and might be curable by any form of treatment.[18]

The Ontario study reviewed more than ten thousand cases. Fifty women were identified as refusing treatment for a variety of reasons. In this group, 70 percent survived for five years after the time of the first symptom. This rate is only a few percentage points lower than the five-year survival rate recorded between 1977 and 1980 by the National Cancer Institute for women who received conventional treatment.

To further illustrate the extremes of possibility in the behavior of cancer, Baum gives examples of two patients with breast cancer. One was a sixty-year-old woman who refused the doctor's recommendation of a radical mastectomy and went on to outlive her doctor and three husbands. At the age of ninety she had "no clinical or radiological evidence of distant dissemination," although she had developed a second tumor in the other breast.

Another woman was forty-five years old and premenopausal. She had no palpable mass; her symptoms consisted of "general discomfort and breathlessness on exertion." Blood-test results indicated anemia and abnormal red and white blood cells. Bone-marrow aspiration confirmed malignancy, and a breast x-ray revealed the location of "three minute foci of cancer." This woman was treated by removal of her ovaries. (Although this may seem a rather peculiar treatment approach, ovaries are a recognized source of estrogen, which stimulates breast-cancer growth. At various times during history, physicians—desperate to find a treatment or treatment combination that would improve survival—have tried everything from inhibiting estrogen production to prescribing estrogen supplements.) There was no mention of any chemotherapy or radiotherapy to the breast during early treatment.

The second woman died eighteen months after her initial consultation. This outcome, in comparison to a woman who did nothing, seems surprising no matter how unusual these examples may be.

TREATMENT OPTIONS

This historical overview made it apparent to me how little really has been learned about breast cancer over the centuries and how minor the improvement in survival has been despite our new treatment protocols. My contemporary options didn't seem considerably more advanced or straightforward than the historical approaches and results I had been reading about.

First I considered surgery. Would there be an advantage to having a lumpectomy? Did I want to have my lymph nodes removed?

My cancer was small (one centimeter) and was considered an infiltrating ductal carcinoma *in situ* (meaning localized in the ducts). But there is no agreement as to how these "early" cancers should be treated. Both extremes—from lumpectomy with close follow-up to removal of both breasts—have been applied to this type and stage of cancer. But long-term follow-up studies are available primarily for mastectomies, although *in situ* cancers are not included in the American Cancer Society incidence rates. They are estimated to constitute an additional 10 to 15 percent.

When my initial biopsy had been done, the surgeon did not get clear margins. Instead he cut into the tumor and, it would seem, spread the cancer cells. I was uncertain whether my immune system could repair this kind of damage. Basically the surgeon had interfered with the body's defense mechanism, which is to create a tumor capsule to corral the problem cells. Partial mastectomy is yet another immune-system-weakening treatment, and evidence suggests that radiotherapy would have adverse effects on the immune system as well.[19]

The basic premise on which I evaluated all treatment options was that my immune system was my most valuable asset for fighting the cancer. To stay true to this conviction, I needed an individualized treatment program. This meant having treatments that were individualized to me, not to the research institute. But my first choice, a lumpectomy without radiation, was met with great resistance by the medical profession because I had a second area in question, which a needle aspiration indicated to be benign.

The consensus leaned toward a mastectomy, since needle aspirations are definitive only when they are positive, indicating cancer, and the doctors didn't want to accept that I just had a mysterious lump. (This lump eventually dissolved on its own and no invasion was ever noted in this tissue, even two years later when my breast was removed.) Although initially it appeared that I had a choice, I was unable to find a surgeon who would perform the surgery I requested. The surgeons felt they would be doing me a "dis-service" to perform such a procedure.

I learned the hard way that breast conservation is not everyone's option, even when the tumor is small. Early small cancers in premenopausal women are treated more aggressively than larger tumors in postmenopausal women because of the estrogen-rich environment premenopausal women provide. The two-step procedure (biopsy, then surgical treatment) gives women an opportunity to feel they are making a choice, but our options are still limited by our surgeons' willingness to cooperate.

Baum points out that although no particular type of treatment has yet proved consistently superior to any other, "as far as survival is concerned, all trials have consistently demonstrated the very poor outlook connected with axillary node involvement." Axillary nodes are the lymph nodes in our armpits. Unfortunately there is no way to determine involvement without removing the lymph nodes, which act as a filtering system for our bodies.

Instinctively, I was opposed to having my lymph nodes removed strictly for diagnostic purposes, and the research I gathered helped me justify my reasoning to the surgeons. I had learned that this was the procedure that most often resulted in postsurgical complications, including edema, restricted mobility, numbness, and potential nerve damage. I had also seen evidence on the usefulness of the lymph nodes as part of a patient's natural resistance to the spread of the cancer. Baum suggests that cancer cells may be able to pass through the lymph nodes without causing damage. He further states that "lymph nodes themselves may be regarded as actively hostile to the proliferation of tumor cells . . . the removal or irradiation of these uninvolved lymph nodes might be potentially harmful to the patient."[20]

Treatment of involved lymph nodes can provide symptomatic relief; however, it is widely accepted as unlikely to positively influence the patient's survival rate. In Baum's discussion of surgery, he states, "New evidence has accumulated suggesting that breast cancer cells gain direct access to the bloodstream and then to the vital organs early in the course of tumor development. Furthermore, tumor cells that reach the lymph nodes are not necessarily trapped there but can either traverse the lymph nodes intact or bypass the lymph nodes via lymphovenous communications."[21]

Current medical opinion is that the lymph nodes are probably not a staging area for further spread of the cancer but rather that an involved axillary node signals, in most instances, that the disease is already systemic.

In the past, doctors believed that when a tumor is in the breast, all breast tissue is affected in both breasts, because the cells do not distinguish between right and left. These old-school surgeons therefore suggested that both breasts be removed to thoroughly treat the cancer. This thinking came from the days when doctors considered breast cancer a local disease. Today it is generally accepted that all breast cancer is systemic, regardless of tumor size, tumor type, or lymph-node status. Since in 1989 the National Cancer Institute recommended chemotherapy for *all* women with any stage of breast cancer, we can reasonably assume that this indicates an acceptance that breast cancer is a systemic disease even at an early stage. The primary purpose of chemotherapy is to "treat not only the visible breast cancer but also any microscopic metastases by giving women cytotoxic drugs that destroy cancer cells."[22]

Treatment for an *in situ* cancer should not necessarily be considered less of a threat because it is small and confined. Although this is an early stage of cancer, it is no less deadly. In hindsight, breast removal is not as outrageous an option as I once thought. This treatment in conjunction with immune-strengthening therapies (which I discuss in depth in Part Two), provides women with an alternative that is least likely to cause new "treatment-induced" cancers.

"I did feel the need to keep some kind of record. Documenting the process photographically accomplished this for me. Body prints were made the night before the operation in response to an intuitive, perhaps irrational, need to ritualize the passage, the impending sense of loss. They commemorate the event with marks that could never be made again."

Margaret Stanton Murray
Corralitos, California

Today, doctors try to recommend lumpectomy and radiation to conserve the breasts (if that is appropriate). A lumpectomy clearly offers a reprieve from amputation, but neither treatment program has demonstrated an improvement in long-term survival. Both these treatments address the local condition only, and radiation is a known carcinogen.

Assuming that I would have my nodes removed and they would prove to be positive, I still had serious reservations about high-dose therapeutic radiation. Was it appropriate? Could my body tolerate the radiation treatments? I had friends who had experienced radiation sickness. Doctors justify radiation therapy as a means of killing the stray cancer cells—but they also kill healthy cells. What are the problems sometimes encountered with radiation?

Mary Spletter, a former cancer patient, writes in *A Woman's Choice: New Options in the Treatment of Breast Cancer* that years after she received five thousand rads of radiation following her mastectomy—solely for preventive therapy against cancer reappearing on her chest wall—she discovered some interesting facts:

> I didn't know that a little more than a year earlier a major study on more than one thousand women from twenty-five institutions had concluded that this treatment really wasn't worthwhile. Women who received radiation did have fewer recurrences of cancer in their armpit and chest wall, but it didn't affect their survival rates any more than if the doctors had treated the recurrences when they appeared.[23]

She adds, "Today [in 1982] there would be near unanimous agreement that I didn't need the radiation. It was easy therapy to go through but it increased the chances that my arm would swell and made my later reconstruction virtually impossible without the addition of new healthy skin." The director of the National Cancer Institute in 1982 confirmed that there is "no reason to offer routine radiation to women after surgery. If nodes contain cancer, you should be put on chemotherapy; if they do not, there is no reason for treatment."[24] It has since become understood that all cells require a blood supply to thrive. Since surgery and scarring diminish the blood flow, chemotherapy (which works via the blood stream) may be less effective in local areas subjected to surgical procedures; therefore radiation is the accepted method of treating these areas.

During the 1980s the NCI returned to supporting the use of radiation after lumpectomy. Treatment approaches seem to be revised with the release of each major study, yet the doctors are emphatic in saying that what they offer is the "state-of-the-art"—that is, the state of *today's* art. Dr. Marc Lipmann, one of the leading breast cancer researchers in the United States, testified before congress on the "state-of-the-art" treatment for breast cancer, saying, "A doctor treating a breast cancer patient is like a caveman trying to stop a speeding car by beating on it with his club."[25]

A patient's geographic location and her choice of hospitals has a great deal to do with the treatment she is offered. Here in Vermont, for example, women who receive radiation treatment have few side effects and little or no skin burning. Yet, a woman in Utah receiving radiation for Stage I node-negative breast cancer received high-dose radiation that

Affix
Postage
Stamp
Here

Inner Traditions International, Ltd.
P.O. Box 388
Rochester, VT 05767

confined her to bed and burned her skin. She was told in 1991 that if this didn't work she could expect to have five years of chemotherapy. This was a highly unusual pronouncement for a Stage I node-negative forty-year-old cancer patient.

Some protocols deliberately seek to "burn" the skin tissue, which results in permanent discoloration and thinning. As in Spletter's case, this high-dose protocol may make the skin unsuitable for reconstruction. Radiation guide marks, or tattoos, are often placed on the patient's chest and can also result in unexpected and permanent skin disfigurement.

Radiation-treatment side effects can appear ten years after treatment and were once considered to be unrelated to breast-cancer treatment. The *British Medical Journal* reported in 1989 that initial evidence pointing to the virtues of radiation therapy in improving recurrence rates did not demonstrate any improvement in mortality, since death may have resulted from other causes related to the therapy itself. Sickness induced by radiation may include heart failure, damage to the myocardium, coronary thrombosis (blood clotting), and new malignancies, some far removed from the radiated site. Although the phenomenon is rare, radiation has been reported to spill to the thyroid, thymus, ribs, the other breast, and lungs and to result in long-term damage from radiation absorption. The *British Medical Journal* notes that patients who were irradiated postoperatively showed "no significant effect on survival up to ten years, but beyond ten years the mortality in the irradiated patients was significantly increased."[26]

These results were most profound for women like myself with early, small breast cancers. We are the women who are being encouraged to utilize "breast conservation surgery" and postoperative radiation, because of the findings of the National Surgical Adjuvant Breast and Bowel Project (NSABP).[27] The Cancer Research Campaign trial concluded that "women with small cancers, perhaps detected by mammography, have an excellent chance of living beyond ten years and would then be at greatest hazard of developing the long-term unwanted effects of radical radiotherapy."[28] (The most widely recognized long-term side effect of radiotherapy is treatment-induced leukemia. "Radical" refers to high-dose therapeutic radiation used with conservation surgery such as a lumpectomy.) The *British Medical Journal,* discussing radiotherapy for ductal carcinoma *in situ* detected by screening, states that in England "radiation is largely restricted to the palliation of symptoms in patients with advanced malignancy or to the cure of those with life-threatening disease for whom other treatment either does not exist or is more toxic."[29]

Women who have a lumpectomy and radiation—the current "gold standard" of treatment—have the same chance for disease-free survival as women who have a mastectomy only (no radiation). But women who have a lumpectomy only (no radiation) have a 37 percent greater chance of a local recurrence after eight years. On this basis, women today generally opt for the less mutilative surgery along with radiation, without fully considering the added risks that radiation therapy involves. What at first glance seems like a straightforward choice—do whatever is necessary to keep our breasts—may result in unanticipated results: permanent skin, size, and color alterations. After radiation treatment, local recurrence may be more difficult to detect—either by physical exam or by mammography—because of scarring and the distortion of the breast tissue.[30] Even the most minimal treatment increases our risk of long-term side effects, future breast cancer, other cancers, or treatment-induced diseases. It will never be as though nothing had happened, no matter how benign the treatment appears.

Joseph Highland describes in *Malignant Neglect* how the medical industry has historically underestimated the dangers of radiation therapy, often being blinded to such an extent that physicians themselves, who were early users, did not take precautions when administering treatments: "In 1944, the *Journal of the American Medical Association* reported that radiologists who worked with x-ray machines on a regular basis were ten times more likely to die from leukemia than other physicians." Now these physicians take precautions and leave the patient alone in the room during treatment. Nonetheless, the history of the radiation-treatment industry repeatedly illustrates that although radiation has at various times been "deemed highly beneficial for large segments of the population," for a multitude of purposes, from enlarged thymus to arthritic disease, years later many of these uses were determined to be dangerous and ineffective.[31]

Doctors and technicians nonetheless continue to express their faith in the safety of today's uses. At least two women I know experienced nausea, diarrhea, and fatigue during their radiation treatments; yet they were told by their physicians that these problems could not be associated with their treatments. When I published a newspaper article in 1989 calling for a closer look into breast-cancer treatment, local radiologists responded by writing letters to the editor denying that radiation has any known harmful side effects.

The dilemma patients must face in deciding whether to undergo radiation treatment for breast cancer involves examining their willingness to accept that the advantages of decreased early recurrence might be offset by the increased risk of getting leukemia, lung cancer, or other treatment-related diseases.

When Dr. Alfred I. Neugut, a cancer researcher at the College of Physicians and Surgeons, Columbia University's medical school in New York, discovered that "women who received radiation treatments for breast cancer are twice as likely to develop lung cancer as breast cancer patients who didn't receive radiation treatments,"[32] he and others attempted to downplay their findings. Neugut is quoted in *The Wall Street Journal* as stating, "the finding [is] mainly of scientific interest and shouldn't alarm women who receive the treatment."

Dr. Samuel Hellman, dean of the University of Chicago Medical School and a radiation therapist who helped pioneer the increasingly popular breast-preservation therapy of lumpectomy plus radiation, attributed these findings to 1970s technology and the angle of the radiation beam, stating that this "has never been a problem before."

Both researchers appear content to reaffirm "that radiation can indeed cause cancer," and willing to discount these rather significant findings in a sample of 56,000 women treated between 1973 and 1986. The study did not address radiation dose and apparently did not draw a comparison between women who were treated with mastectomy and radiation (less common in the 1970s unless the disease had advanced beyond the breast tissue) and women who elected to undergo lumpectomy and radiation (the treatment that gained widespread acceptance during this time period).

I was an unusual patient in that I declined the recommendation of radiotherapy, and I found that the doctors were surprised by the health of my breast tissue even two and a half years after my diagnosis. Reconstruction remained a viable option for me at all stages because the breast skin tissue had not been damaged by previous radiation treatment.

After becoming convinced that radiation therapy was not for me, I turned my attention to chemotherapy. I understood and accepted the premise that breast cancer is a systemic disease at any stage, so I could see why chemotherapy was promoted for treating early-stage breast cancers. Studies evaluating the effectiveness of therapies, however, demonstrate that chemotherapy offers no fewer risks and no less ambiguity in its results than do radiation or surgery.

Dr. Samuel Broder, director of the National Cancer Institute, acknowledged in 1990: "The national cancer statistics for mortality rates from breast cancer have hardly changed over the last fifteen years in spite of the triumphal attitudes of the American medical oncology." In the same statement he went on to admit that although "adjuvant systemic therapy [chemotherapy] can perturb the natural history of breast cancer by having a profound influence on time to relapse, the results, expressed as overall reduction in mortality rates, are so modest that there must be something wrong with the prevailing biologic model."[33] Essentially, the director of one of the world's largest cancer institutes is saying that perhaps we are barking up the wrong tree.

A recent report by the Government Accounting Office (GAO) states that the number of breast-cancer patients receiving chemotherapy has increased 300 percent since 1975. The results, however, do not demonstrate a proportionate improvement in long-term mortality. In fact, the patients reviewed who didn't undergo chemotherapy lived as long as those who took the treatment.[34]

> The standard Milan CMF [cyclophosphamide, methotresate, and fluorouracil] adjuvant chemotherapy regimen for patients with operable breast cancer and histologically positive axillary nodes indicates overall survival as CMF 50 percent, versus controls without chemotherapy of 38 percent.[35]

The report actually goes on to say that "while these data are encouraging, they also demonstrate that at least 60 percent of the treated patients will still die of their breast cancer with first generation adjuvant therapy." Reading these percentages may appear as though someone made a mistake, but I attribute this to medical double-talk. What initially appears to be the result isn't in fact the long-term result.

The current success rate of chemotherapy in treating breast cancer is a three percent improvement in three-year survival, between 1975 and 1983. David Ginsburg and associates from the Kingston Regional Cancer

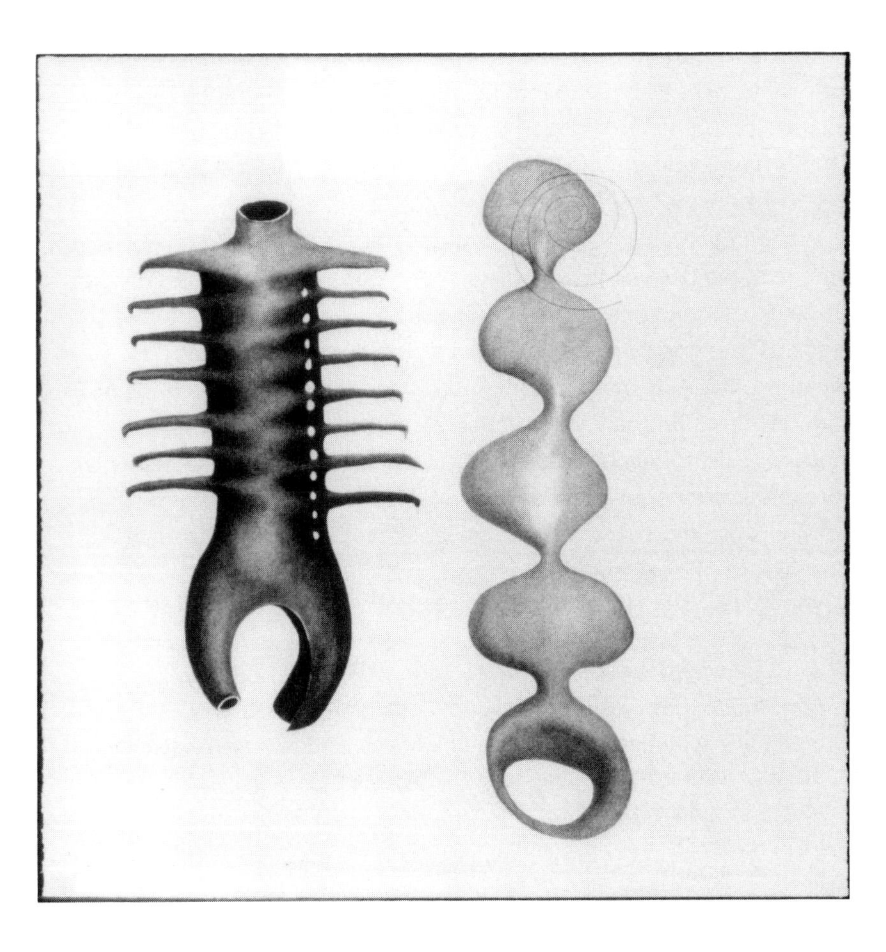

Untitled
Charma Le Edmonds, Bethesda, Maryland
Charcoal on paper, 42" x 42", unframed, 1993

"It is so hard to accept the words, 'It's malignant,' and the next words, 'I recommend a mastectomy in your case due to the aggressiveness of cancer in young women.' Then there was a heavy pause. 'The baby won't survive the surgery and the chemotherapy.'"

Centre in Ontario, Canada, state, "The recent advice from the U.S. National Cancer Institute recommending the use of chemotherapy for all patients, including node-negative, does not seem to be justified. The benefits have been modest and may not outweigh the cost and toxic effects of such therapy."[36]

When I eventually had surgery and learned that five lymph nodes were involved, I asked my oncologist for a copy of the statistics on the follow-up treatment he was recommending. He offered the "study standards"—a comprehensive review of the drugs to be tested—for CAF (cyclophosphamide, adriamycin, flourouracil) activated March 22, 1991. (Many different protocols are available for chemotherapy, and study standards exist for each protocol.) Although this document contains far more information than most patients wish to read or can comprehend, it also spells out short- and long-term side effects in a sample patient consent form. For example:

> Doxorubicin (adriamycin) may cause a lowering of the blood cell and platelet counts (which could cause an increased risk of infection, easy bruising, and bleeding), nausea and vomiting, hair loss, discolored urine (pink), darkening of the nail beds, and skin rashes. Should this drug leak from my vein during administration I could experience severe skin damage similar to a burn. At higher cumulative doses than I will receive in this program, adriamycin can cause symptomatic heart failure, which may be permanent. Symptoms of heart failure include shortness of breath, decreased exercise tolerance, and swollen ankles. This is usually prevented by stopping the drug before it reaches a dangerous level. Other complaints include fatigue, mouth sores, and liver abnormalities.[37]

Adriamycin represents one of six drugs included in this protocol. Other drugs in addition to those contained in the study standards might be required to lessen side effects such as toxicity, nausea, and diarrhea.

The *Lancet* on August 23, 1986, discussed the "Mechanism of Action of Adjuvant Chemotherapy in Early Breast Cancer," stating that CMF "in early breast cancer prolongs relapse-free survival and overall survival in premenopausal patients, but has only a slight effect in postmenopausal patients."[38] These findings may have influenced the recommendations by the National Institutes of Health consensus panel on breast-cancer therapy. The panel recommended that postmenopausal women with the disease be given hormonal therapy (tamoxifen) and that some younger women who had not yet reached menopause be treated with chemotherapy.

Both chemotherapy and tamoxifen can cause drug-induced early menopause or menopause-like symptoms in premenopausal women, resulting in yet another set of problems that range from hot flashes and night sweats to heart disease and osteoporosis. Tamoxifen, which has been in use since the 1970s, has also been observed to cause irregular menses, vaginal discharge and dryness, nausea, retinal changes, thrombosis, and endrometrial cancers. Because of such side effects, doctors have not always been eager to prescribe tamoxifen; however, this seems to be changing. Currently women of all ages and stages at diagnosis are being encouraged to take tamoxifen, the latest "wonder" drug.

The most recently acclaimed study by the Early Breast Cancer Trialists' Collaborative Group, headed by Richard Peto, studied 17,000 women with early breast cancer. The study noted that the probability of women surviving ten years was 50 percent in the women who took tamoxifen, compared with a 42 percent survival in women who had not taken tamoxifen.[39]

Doctors compelled by such statistics then face the dilemma of deciding who will benefit most from these high-risk treatments. Since some patients with node-negative estrogen-receptive tumors still experience relapse, scientists continue to search for some definitive marker to predict relapse or cure as well as determine the need for chemotherapy. Staging and grading are considered classical prognostic markers.

The most sophisticated breast cancer therapies offered by the medical profession today provide mixed results that have necessitated conducting more and more tests and clinical trials. Every few years the protocols (prescribed treatments) are changed, so no one can really say at the time a new treatment is offered whether it will perform better or worse than the treatments it replaces.

Staging is used to give doctors a bench mark for discussing treatment options and survival rates. Grading is a more recent and complex technique for predicting the likelihood of a relapse and need for aggressive forms of treatment. These markers remain limited in their predictive value, but a woman may want to explore the appropriateness of the various tests available with her doctor, before the biopsy is complete.

New yet still imprecise indicators include measurement of DNA content, S-phase fraction, HER-2 amplification or overexpression, and Cathepsin D.[40] All these tests require that the doctor obtain adequate tissue for pathology analysis.

Initially it was so difficult for me to talk about my cancer that it would have been impossible for me to make a truly informed decision. My gut-level reaction to my diagnosis was that radiation and chemotherapy were not viable options for me. The information I had gathered served to reinforce this feeling. I was extremely drug sensitive, beyond anything that doctors were willing to acknowledge, and the risks involved with radiation were too great. I also decided that if I had to have a mastectomy and lose my left breast, I would prefer to have both removed. Balance is very important to me.

When I told my doctor about my thoughts, these ideas were met with as much opposition as my request for a lumpectomy without radiation. *The only way I could get the doctors' approval was to do exactly what they wanted.*

Although we can't know initially which type of breast cancer—intraductal, invasive, or lobular—we have, a needle aspiration or biopsy will usually provide this information. As I became armed with information about the odds, risks, and uniqueness of my type of cancer, and about how my prognostic risk factors were intertwined with variables such as my age, I evaluated and reevaluated my choices about treatment many times. At every stage I knew I could only base my decision on the best information available, and I expected the same of my doctors.

This information provided me with the lifeline I needed to feel I was doing everything possible to stay alive. The facts forced me to be objective and confront my fears. Once I accepted that the worst that could happen was that I would die, no matter who made the final treatment decision, I also realized that the doctors didn't have any special tricks or wisdom to significantly change the course of this disease. My future really did depend on me.

ART TWO:

earching for Cure

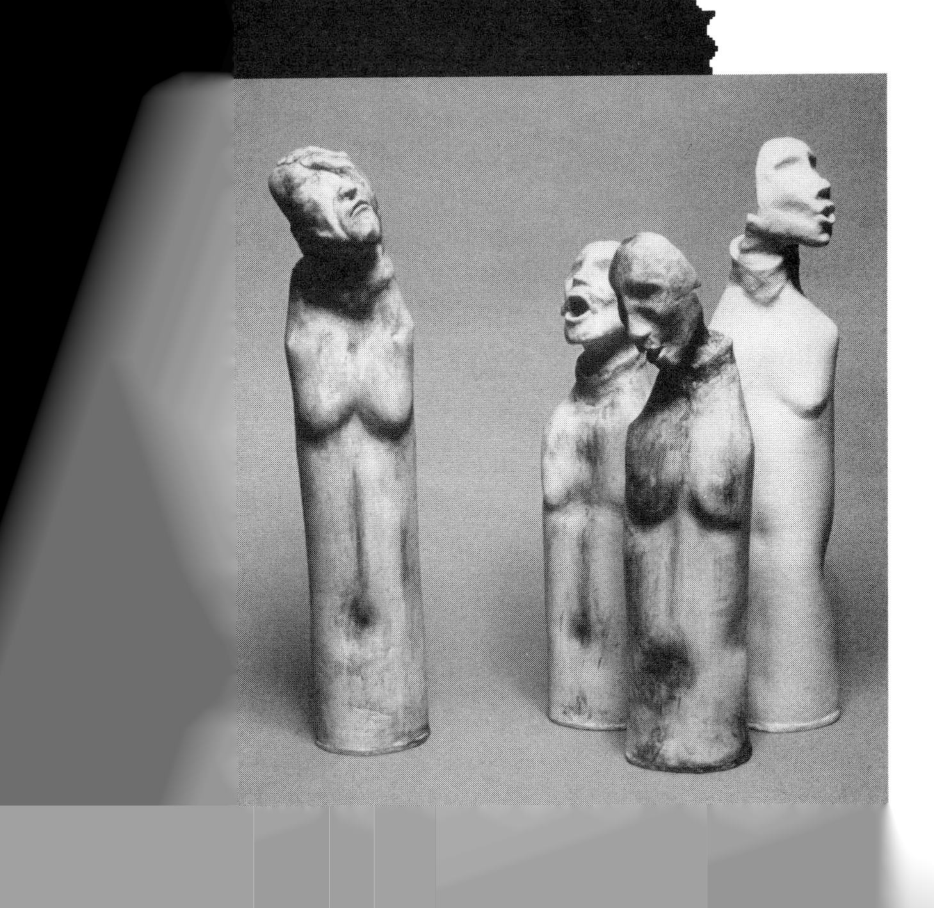

"When the nightmare confronts you, you want to scream, but can't. The scream might convey your feeling, but it's locked inside your head, horrifically echoing one word: NO! Two years after the mastectomy, I had an uncontrollable belief that I could draw, although I never had before. I took a few art classes, touched clay, and suddenly, I was able to say what no words were adequate to express for me. I was breathing very thin air, and the better part of my intellect and spirituality were open to exploration."

Grief Masks I–IV
Paulette Carr, St. Louis, Missouri
Porcelain and Stains, 24"h x 28"w x 20"d, 1989

4

Women's Spirituality

If you tell a lie, you lose part of your conscience. If you continue to lie you will have no conscience left.

A wise woman

Healing, and arriving at a place to heal, require an opening up to that which is beyond this realm. In this place there is no language and many spirits. Doctors call mysterious, unexplainable healing "spontaneous remission." New Agers might describe these occasions as transformational. Believers will say that when they were touched by the hand of the Lord they were healed.

Having cancer is a "remarkable event." Scientists and engineers use this term to describe an unexpected occurrence in the nuclear-power industry. Discovering breast cancer is unexpected; what can happen after the diagnosis is indeed remarkable; and both can be catastrophic.

What happens to those of us who experience having cancer is very difficult to describe. Eleanor Ott, Ph.D., who specializes in folklore, remarks, "Mysteries cannot be spoken about, only experienced." Sig Lonegren, an expert on sacred sites, describes "gnowing" as being able to sense—knowing for himself because he has tasted the other side. Both Ott and Lonegren are talking about the energies of the earth and the mysteries of life. Both know these kinds of experiences, but neither has had a life-threatening illness like breast cancer.

Sometimes an illness like breast cancer can catapult a person to "the edge," as described by Ross Jennings, founder of the Dancing Dragon Center for the Art of Placement in New Hampshire:

THE EDGE

I am the edge of darkness
Where light arises
I am the light that shines from the darkness
I am the darkness that engenders the light.
Light and darkness weaving
That is my becoming.
I am the nowness of that becoming
I am that which becomes
I am that.
I crossed the edge of darkness
And there I met the light
And in the light saw darkness dying
As it birthed the light.
Light's seed of darkness finds fulfillment
In the newborn light.
Oh, light! Remember the womb that bore thee
For if you are to be reborn you first must die.
If you are to be remembered you first must be forgotten.
Light in darkness dying, sleep forgetful sleep.
Life's first movement is a forgetting
And in completion is remembrance.
Return to the source that you may rise anew.
To fulfill the Earth is spirit's dying
But die it must to be reborn.
We must face that which we've averted open and empty stand.
Let only love flow through you
Forgiveness is the grace we are given.
Accept, unite, and with the Earth's fire rising
Know that only you can birth a star!

Illness can help us see how fine the line is between light and dark, how dark is not always bad or evil, and how through this experience we can learn things we have not necessarily been educated about. It is a time when reason may have to be set aside, science can become too limiting, and accessing a higher realm can seem very appropriate.

This might be just the kind of personal crisis needed to go beyond the *me* to seeing the *we*. We are not alone, we are not in charge, and our whole world can't be controlled by what we do or say. There is more to life than us humans.

As a child I always had a strong belief in God, although my religious training and my family's religious beliefs were scattered and undirected at best. My family did not follow a strict doctrine but rather raised us to be interested in religion in a more philosophical sense.

My belief in God came from somewhere else. It was internal and very much a part of me. I found comfort in my knowing, but I didn't feel any obligation to worship. Yet it was something I would turn to at a time of crisis.

When my cancer was diagnosed, turning inward for answers seemed automatic. My tools became yoga, meditation, affirmations, visualization, dowsing, and a relationship with God. I asked to see the cancer in me—to see where it came from, what controlled it, and what caused it. I asked for assistance in making the difficult decisions that needed to be made. I asked to be led to books and articles that I should read and to people I needed to meet. I asked for my cancer to be taken away, for my breast to be spared, and for information about how I should use my experience. I placed my life in the hands of God and asked for his guidance.

I discovered that what was happening in my life was not an accident, a coincidence, or a result of chance. This was an experience I would learn from and be guided through. I realized I had to work to stay open to this opportunity. If I numbed myself with drugs, alcohol, food, or other compensation I might miss this important lesson—one that I did not choose but still had a choice about.

Once I decided to accept the oneness of my cancer and me, I decided to love my tumor because it was a part of me. This very dark moment also became an incredibly light time. I came in touch with my higher self, my more spiritual self, as I never had before. I learned to trust my intuition, to believe in myself, and to stand up for what I believed. I felt cleansed from having started a macrobiotic diet within ten days of my diagnosis. This cleaning out of the tissue toxins was supported by daily visualization and yoga practice, which seemed to be a natural extension of my new diet.

What transpired was completely unexpected. For the first time, I had to bring who I was to what needed to be accomplished. It was no longer an option to turn over my problem or my life to someone else—in this case, the doctor. Myself, my being, my body—all were intricately intertwined. This disease wasn't out there somewhere; it was inside. The cancer was not an invader; it was my own cells malfunctioning. The cure offered to me by the doctors could not selectively remove the bad cells without destroying some of the good, and both were part of me. I felt that if I made the cancer my enemy, I would be turning against myself.

Nonetheless, my thoughts and emotions weren't a single stream of wanting to embrace my disease. There were also times when I wanted to see action. I wanted to see some results for all the time I was investing in my healing. I wanted to be reassured that what I was doing could make me well. On some days I would fall into the old patterns of expecting to see quick results. I had had a great deal of experience with achieving the goals I set out to accomplish. My favorite saying was "Find a need and fill it." Like the child who says, "Mommy, I'm cold"—and whose mother responds, "Here, honey, put on your sweater"—I had days when I quietly wished for easy solutions for my breast cancer. It would be so straightforward if, after they detected it, the doctors could just make it go away.

Yet, I kept coming back to the phrase "This time there are no simple answers." It didn't matter whether the answer was surgery, chemotherapy, radiation, or all three. It didn't matter whether the tumor was only a one-centimeter tumor with no lymph nodes involved, because other women with this same diagnosis were still having recurrences and dying.

Although I felt little support for my quest from society in general, I also discovered I was not alone in my pursuits. Someone was always there to help me as I wrestled with this foreign and amorphous process. My therapist, who joined me two weeks after my diagnosis; my macrobiotic counselor, whom I discovered after only five days of eating this new way; new friends; and writers of books about mystical experiences all helped me traverse this new path. This path had numerous obstacles that I had to prepare for. Some required that I find a way to dissolve the obstacle; others required that I confront it, recognize it, and even love it. Each obstacle carried a unique message for me in solving this health-building puzzle.

Dan Millman, author of *Way of the Peaceful Warrior,* was this kind of guide. He helped me look at my anger as I read: "Neither resolutions nor understanding will ever make you strong. Resolutions have sincerity, logic has clarity; but neither has the energy you will need. Let *anger* [emphasis added] be your resolution, your logic."[1] Expressing my anger about having breast cancer when I was only thirty-eight years old, sharing it in writing class, and allowing it to be seen in front of people I hardly knew helped me learn to use my anger rather than suppress or deny it.

I realized that everything that had already happened in my life would have an influence on how I approached this new challenge. My family and friends were like the vertebrae in my back. The whole cast of characters made up my ability to stand erect and to be. How I viewed my life experiences related to how flexible or stiff I had become with age. I learned to apply and learn from my past experience rather than treat this crisis as isolated and separate.

My meditation time was like a microscope. I was the observer. I didn't need to dictate the next step, just to observe and report the status. I kept a daily journal about events as they transpired. I believed that having an understanding of myself, my being, would be the first step toward my own healing. I would hear a voice inside me telling me that the reason I got cancer was really to discover health, balance, and harmony—the kind of harmony that cannot be achieved with drugs that treat symptoms. I experienced foods and homeopathic remedies, body adjustment and cleansing—all in an attempt to achieve a better balance and clear thinking. I watched and listened to how my body responded and then adjusted my program until I found which combinations worked best for me.

The more I let meditation be my observatory, the more God became my guide. I asked for help, then I waited and watched. My first indication that something different was happening was when I could see that there were more than two short and uncertain paths for healing. The doctor said there were only two choices: follow the prescribed treatment or die. Through prayer and meditation I discovered a third option, one that looked much longer. This path didn't aggressively attack the cancer or my body; instead, it worked on strengthening my immune system. I believed the miracle serum was in my body. I was capable of producing it, but first my body had to be restored to a healthier condition. And I discovered this path was longer in two ways. First, the healing took longer and required more patience and self-absorption. Second, it would lead to long-term health instead of a short-term fix.

Six months after I started the macrobiotic diet and this spiritual and biomedical investigation, the sign I had been asking for occurred. The lump in the lower right quadrant of my left breast dissolved.

I had been able to observe the lump changing form and position during my visualization time. It was no longer hard, and it seemed to move around on its own. These observations were confirmed by touch and by mammograms. Originally the lump was at seven o'clock, but without any noticeable event it would move to nine o'clock and back again. My visualization involved looking inside my body, looking inside my breast and my lymph nodes. I looked at the inside as if my eyes were attached to some kind of inner probe. I could examine these different areas and draw pictures of what I saw. I watched the cell activity and the tissue.

When I observed this particular mass and compared it to the area that had been biopsied, I could see that there was no physical connection between the two areas. But in the early stages of my visualization practice I felt strongly that this lump was still a significant threat. I believed it was at the stage where the cells can grow into a malignant tumor or be transformed back to a benign tumor. Nevertheless, I believed that because I could see it, I could dissolve it myself. My oncologist didn't have this same confidence. While I continued my meditation practices she became very concerned about the changes and requested I have a second mammogram. When the mammogram came back showing a cyst-like mass, she insisted that I get a biopsy. After four months, my meditation and visualization were both indicating that the tumor was no longer a threat. But the surgeon who had taken over my case remained emotionally removed and skeptical about my desire to heal myself.

He asked me in an academic manner, "What do you think is happening?"

"I think that I have lost a great deal of weight due to the change in my diet, but the lump feels as though it is the same size, although my breasts are smaller now."

He decided to measure the lump and compare the results to what had been recorded during my initial visit. "It's two centimeters, same as before. What do you want me to do about it?"

I told him that my oncologist was very concerned because the lump had changed since the initial mammogram. "I'm willing to have it removed," I told him. "But I believe it's benign because of the way it looks on the mammogram. It's like a little ball of jelly. That's what a benign tumor looks like, isn't it?"

"It could mean that, but we can't be sure with your history of prior malignancy."

"When could you remove it?" I asked

"I'll have to have the nurse check my schedule. She has gone for the day. I'll have her call you tomorrow."

This visit took place around six o'clock on a Wednesday evening. The nurse called me at eight the following morning. "We have scheduled you for surgery at noon today. Report to outpatient check-in half an hour early." I was startled by the short notice, but felt it was time to have this little thing removed. I expected only the best results.

I arranged a ride and arrived at the hospital as instructed. By the time I had completed all the forms and made my way up to the floor where the operating room was located, it was noon. I was greeted by the same two nurses who had attended my first biopsy. It was like a homecoming. They were very friendly and expressed concern about me and my treatment choices. I appreciated their interest, even though I felt a little like the sheep who had strayed from the flock.

The surgeon entered the room, scrubbed and ready to perform. I was already on the table, with my one breast sterile and exposed to his view. He palpated my left breast to locate the lump. It had been easily detected only eighteen hours earlier, but now he couldn't find it.

"Put your arm up. Now down. Now up. I think I found it. Now down. Well, maybe you'll have to keep it up." The doctor probed, and finally after several minutes he removed his gloves and tried to locate it with his bare hands.

I joked about how funny it was—after all this time that he had been trying to get me on the operating table, now the lump had disappeared.

I'm sure my humor about this situation was partially caused by my nervousness. But the doctor remained serious. He simply could not believe this was possible.

They sterilized me again. The doctor scrubbed and put on a new set of gloves. Then he said, "Okay, I've found it. I'm ready." He applied a local anesthesia and made his cut.

"Doctor!" I exclaimed involuntarily. "Why so large?" The nurse turned to me in amazement and adjusted her glasses, as though perhaps I could see a reflection. Then she asked me, "Did you feel that?"

I couldn't explain it intellectually. I "saw" the incision. It was larger than I had expected it needed to be. When the nurse spoke to me I attempted to make sense of what I knew I couldn't know. I had been anesthetized, and I really couldn't *feel* it, but trying to reason this out confused me further.

I had experienced what people describe as an "out of body" experience. I was both on the operating table and floating above it, watching the operation. My alarm was justified and accurate. The surgeon later explained that since he had not been able to find the lump, he made the incision to obtain a cross section so he could see what was happening.

The lump had apparently dissolved during the night. And the surgeon, in total disbelief that this was possible, violated my trust in him. He chose to perform unauthorized exploratory surgery to satisfy his own curiosity. It was not until after the surgery was over that he informed me that he did not remove the lump. And it was not until I removed the bandages that I discovered that the incision was in a different location than I had expected—at nine o'clock and across the center of my breast.

When I asked for an explanation, he said he had just removed some tissue because "if it was malignant, you know what that means."

I said, "No, what?"

"It means you'll lose your whole breast anyway."

When the doctor came into the waiting room shortly after surgery, he said that the initial pathology report indicated that the tissue was normal. There were no cancer cells. I felt vindicated. I had proved that my body was capable of repairing itself.

Two weeks later, however, I went to the hospital and requested a copy of the written pathology report for my records. This report was different from the surgeon's verbal report. It indicated that cancer was detected. What was even more shocking was that this report had been placed in my file, yet the doctor's office had never contacted me about the different results. Instead, the surgeon wrote a follow-up written report for my file recommending a mastectomy. The location of the biopsy was incorrectly noted to correspond with his earlier reports.

The area of the second biopsy or the disappearing lump never developed any further problems. The lump never returned, and when I did have a mastectomy, twenty-two months later, because of a recurrence at the site of the initial biopsy, the pathology report indicated that no cancer cells existed in this area. My cancer had remained localized to the upper outer quadrant, the location of the first biopsy.

Even though my intuitive sense had been there to aid me, I failed to trust it. I wanted scientific confirmation. I consented to, and paid for, surgery that was completely unnecessary—surgery that only created confusion and doubt. This was one of those times when the scientific and spiritual paths didn't mix. I was on one path, and yet I attempted to use another system to prove to myself that what I was doing was working. The scientific model had no tolerance for the possibility of a miracle, so science was applied in a dishonest way. To this day I believe a false report was created to cover the surgeon's tracks.

There is truly a kind of seeing that goes beyond the seeing we do with our eyes. This kind of seeing is difficult to admit to other people. At times it is difficult to admit to ourselves. It is not considered natural or normal to see with more than our eyes. But we can. The blind see this way, and I think I too developed the ability to see this way perhaps because I had a serious visual problem as a child. This type of seeing, which Lonegren calls "gnowing," is how I helped myself heal. It also helped me develop many of my theories about breast cancer.

I saw in my cells that there was a link between many of the factors that are suspected to contribute to breast cancer. During a spiritual experience I saw this link coming from the center of my brain, directly behind my eyes. I have since learned that this area of the brain is called the hypothalamus, which is in fact the control center for the nervous (electrical) and endocrine (chemical) systems. A simple anatomy book helped me match my visualizations to an illustrated representation (figure 2, page 70). I had never studied anatomy, so I wasn't immediately able to label this location or its known function. The relevance of this image

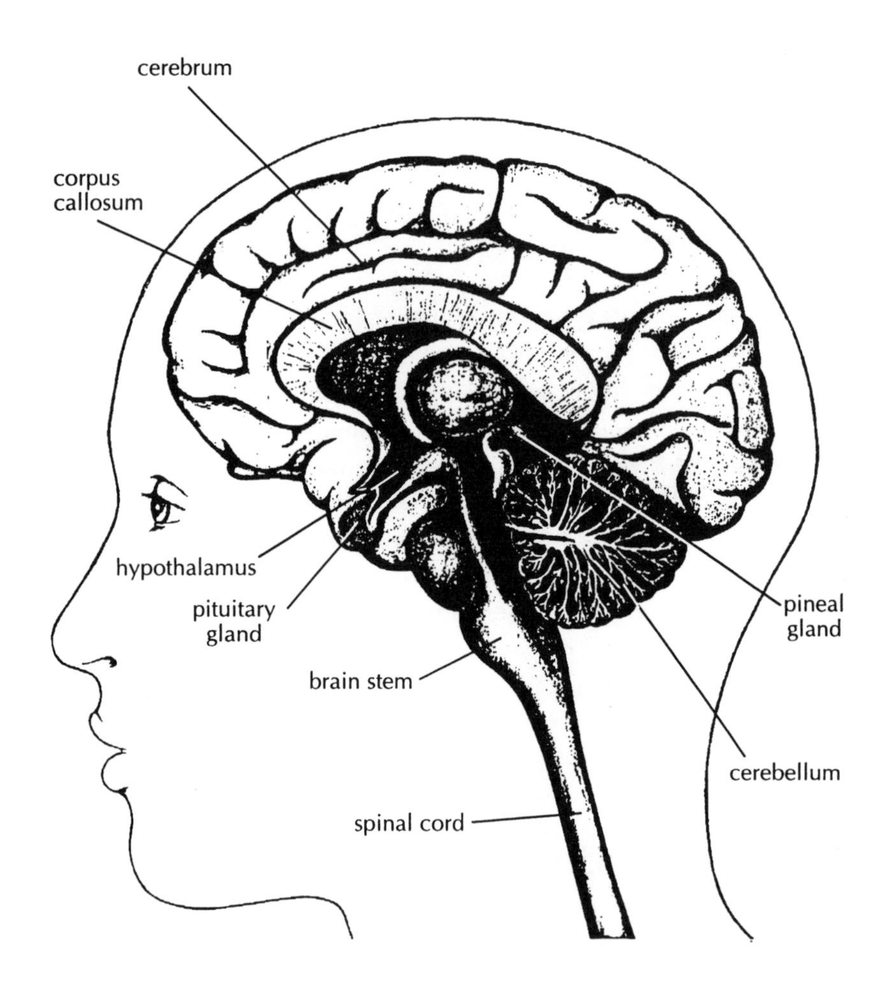

FIGURE 2

CROSS-SECTION OF BRAIN SHOWING HYPOTHALAMUS

From Ruth Dowling Bruun, M.D., and Bertel Bruun, M.D., *The Human Body* (New York: Random House Library, 1982).

came when I started to piece together what I was intuiting with what I was learning at the library. Cancer, particularly breast cancer, was a subject that I knew nothing about, and had no background in, yet it unfolded for me as if I were following a carefully designed course outline. One week I was researching the hypothalamus, the next week the endocrine system, and the next the female reproductive system.

I felt as though I were being led to study particular hormones—hormones I had never heard of—for a reason. Our hormones are regulated by the hypothalamus as well, in a complex "feedback loop" that engages the pituitary and the pineal glands in working to maintain homeostasis (the body's steady state). Homeostasis involves both the chemical and physical conditions of our body: temperature, hunger, digestion, urination, sugar and calcium levels, the ability to stay upright (like a "gravity meter"), moisture and thirst, breathing, responsiveness to light, and healing of wounds. Our hormones are responsible for governing the speed and reaction of these body functions. Before beginning my investigation, I thought that hormones were only for reproduction. I was familiar mainly with estrogen and progesterone. Now I would be exposed to the "symphony of hormones" that regularly send chemical messages throughout our bodies.

Questions seemed to be posed by my invisible inner teacher on one day, then I investigated the answers until I had an understanding of that aspect of the problem. I followed these clues and later integrated the answers into an elaborate healing plan for myself, a plan that was based as much on scientific data as on spiritual guidance. I required confirmation for what I was being led to see and to know. I was unwilling to just accept the spiritual teachings without substantial medically documented background. No matter how much more information I demanded to know, I continued to be led to the right periodicals, books, and experts. Each contained one part, and none had the complete solution.

My inner guidance helped me realize that women have a powerful interconnectedness with the earth. We have monthly cycles that can be influenced by the sun and the moon. We have hormones that are delicately balanced to create perfect homeostasis. Our physical and mental health can be affected by the seasons, by drugs, and by electromagnetic fields. When we are ill, when we cannot reach homeostasis, then this is perhaps a statement about the condition of humanity.

While writing the chapter "Strengthening the Immune System" I had a dream. I think dreams can sometimes reveal what we are trying to comprehend. Understanding my role in my healing was one question I could not resolve.

So here's my dream, and perhaps the answer, from my subconscious to yours:

> Four thugs (wearing black leather jackets) were taking my friends and me down to the beach. We thought we were all going on a picnic. It was late in the afternoon and we were in four cars. When we got out of the cars, I suddenly somehow realized they were going to rape us.
>
> There was a long strip of shops close to the beach, and as soon as the cars were parked and everyone was gathering together the picnic stuff, I bolted away and ran into a nearby drugstore.
>
> I was frantic, screaming, "Call the police! These guys are going to rape us down by the beach." The sales clerk looked at me calmly and asked, "What guys? Where are they? How do you know they are going to rape you?"
>
> I could see I wasn't getting anywhere, so I ran out of the drugstore and into the card shop.
>
> "Help me! Call the police! These guys are going to rape me and my friends." A woman asked, "How many of you are there? Why do you think they are going to rape you?" I ran out of the card shop and into a pet store.
>
> "Call the police! There are some rapists who have tried to attack my friends and me." Another woman looked at me numbly. "What did they do? Can you explain their behavior?"
>
> No one would believe me. Here I was crazy out of my mind with fear and they were asking for details.

I suddenly woke up.

I decided that what my dream was trying to tell me was that women's intuition is often not trusted, sometimes not even by women themselves. We have been conditioned to follow the male model of analytical reasoning. We buy into male standards of quantifying our perceptions with facts and figures, all the while abandoning our personal stories and inner voice. This has become society's standard for measuring appropriate rational behavior. The more we are educated in fields like law or science, the more we become indoctrinated into this kind of thinking. "If it can't be analyzed it isn't so" is the bottom line.

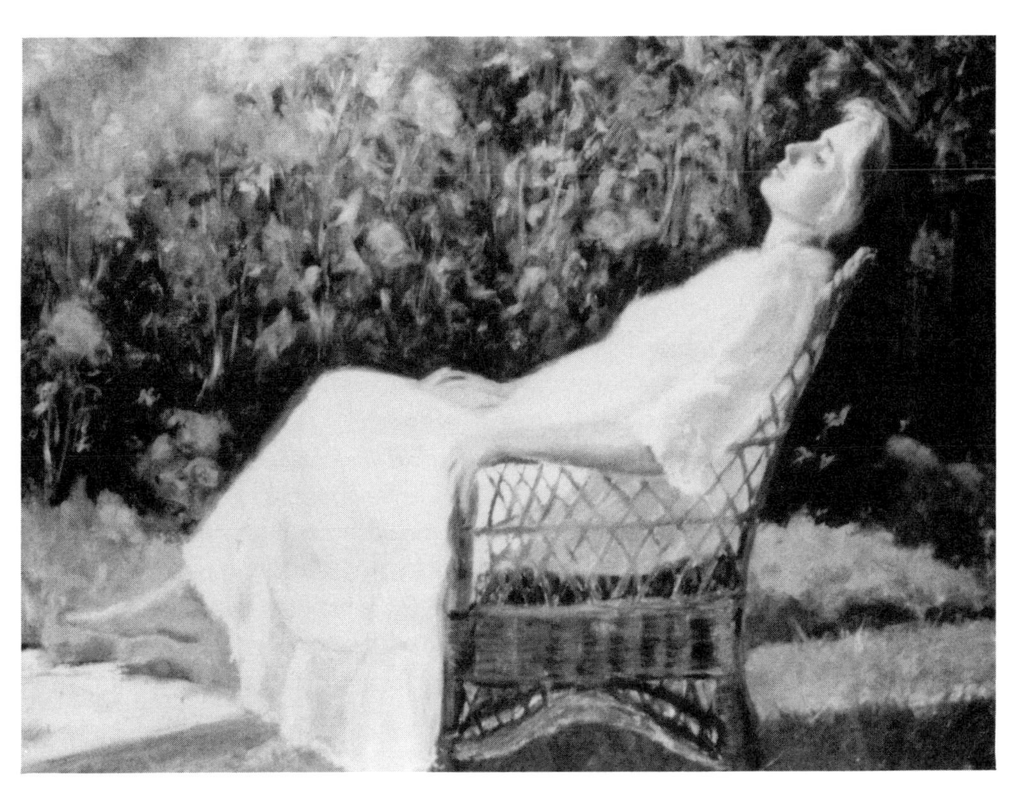

Psalm 23
Sarah Kagan, Easton, Maryland
Oil on canvas, 30" x 36", 1986

"Seven years ago I had breast cancer. My right breast was removed. I sat down and had a good cry and then got on with my life."

We are different because we are women. In recorded history, this difference has been portrayed as inferior and dangerous in spite of the fact that ancient and prehistoric cultures revered and deified women as life-givers. It is only today that women are beginning to reclaim, acknowledge, and celebrate our uniqueness and our intuitiveness. Women as the world's visionaries must be saved to save our planet.

I have heard of other people faced with life-threatening illness who experienced both voices and visions and who interpreted these experiences as a sign that they were dying. At times I too had fears that my unusual experiences might indicate a nearness to the time when I would cross over into the spiritual world. I realize now that the voices and visions were, at all times, trying to assist me, not trying to take me.

One morning I was awakened very early by a message that kept repeating over and over in my mind, "I give myself permission to have a life-threatening illness, then to be well." The message would not stop, so I turned on the light and wrote it down in my journal. I then turned off the light, fluffed my pillow, adjusted the covers, and attempted to doze off again. No sooner had I gone through these motions than another message began to play in my mind: "I see an enlightened understanding of myself as a result of my illness." I could not get the new message to stop until I turned on the light and wrote it down. As soon as I wrote one message down, a new one presented itself until—almost two hours later—I had twelve messages.

I finally went back to sleep. When I awoke in the morning and reread the messages, I marveled at their wisdom and completeness. The experience was quite different from a dream—or even from my meditations—and I haven't had an experience like it since. However, I understod that I was to share the messages with others. I found that I could use them as life affirmations, choosing whichever one I was drawn to at a given moment and repeating it over and over again. Each message carries a key that unlocked a door deep in my own psyche. I'm grateful for the opportunity to pass them on to you.

TWELVE STEPS TO WELL-BEING

1. I give myself permission to have a life-threatening illness, then to be well.
2. I see an enlightened understanding of myself as a result of my illness.

3. I am willing to place my wellness above all else.
4. I have become open to changes of all kinds.
5. I am a powerful being of light.
6. As I open new channels, insights will be revealed to me.
7. Having a life-threatening illness is my opportunity to discover health.
8. I accept my illness as life threatening.
9. The area of my body where my illness chose to manifest itself is with purposefulness.
10. The prescription for wellness is choosing to be in harmony with nature.
11. Being one with nature occurs for all living things.
12. The sources of this disease, of change, and of wellness are God's choice.

5

Strengthening the Immune System

Physical sciences have advanced far beyond the simple mechanics of the sixteenth and seventeenth centuries. Most of medicine, on the other hand, is still stuck in the old concept of the body as a system of pumps and pulleys, pipes and fluids.

Annemarie Colbin, *Food and Healing*

The doctor of the future will give no medicine, but will interest his patient in the care of the human frame, in diet and in the cause and prevention of disease.

Thomas A. Edison

My immune system became my yardstick for weighing all my health-restoring decisions—including the use of alternative treatment programs.

The questions I would ask were these: Would this treatment strengthen or weaken my immune system? What would be the condition of my existing and new cells after the treatment? Could I remove the old toxins that I was storing in my cells, without feeding the cancer? Would the cancer grow at a rate more rapid than my ability to clean up my cell environment?

Cancer is systemic in both our bodies and our lives. Therefore, the concept of a "quick fix" had to be eliminated from my treatment expectations. Speaking to others about their treatment experience, with both traditional and nontraditional techniques, helped me set realistic expectations for my own treatment. I knew from the beginning that this was not something that the doctors could just make go away. I wanted to participate in my treatment—and I discovered that any method of restoring my health was likely to be a long, slow process. Furthermore, I believed that my recovery could be influenced by my body's ability to respond to the new environment I would be providing.

Our different systems—the immune system, the endocrine system, the central nervous system—all function together in the body like instruments making up a symphony orchestra. Talking about the endocrine system as if it were totally separate and isolated from the nervous system, for instance, is far too mechanistic and simplistic. Cancer is a disorder of all our systems. To correct this disorder, all our systems need to be strengthened.

Fighting my breast cancer not only involved eliminating the tumor and the potentially lethal cells in my bloodstream but also involved avoiding new exposures to carcinogenic, "cancer-promoting" substances. Initially this task seemed impossible. Many cancer specialists believe that the environment may contribute as much as 70 to 90 percent to the risk factor of developing cancer.[1]

Evidence indicates that in the past, diseases came under control through prevention rather than through cure.[2] How was prevention achieved? Some researchers suggest that a better diet, improved hygiene, and a more favorable relationship between microorganisms and humans were major contributors to these trends, with better nutrition accounting for three-fourths of the effect.[3] Our twentieth-century lifestyle is literally filled with cancer-causing substances—PCBs, DDT, and DDE are just a few toxins that have actually been observed in the tissue of women with breast cancer. One study found that levels of these "hormone mimicking" substances were 50 to 60 percent higher in women who were biopsied and determined to have breast cancer.[4] While authors of this study did not attempt to identify the source of these toxins, another study did.

Two researchers recently investigated why Israel's breast-cancer mortality rates dropped 8 percent between 1976 and 1986, even though the overall increase in risk factors during this period would seemingly have resulted in an increase in deaths. The risk factors examined included fat intake (which had increased among Isreali population by 19 percent), fruit and vegetable intake (decreased by 3 percent), cereal intake (decreased by 8 percent), alcohol and total calorie intake (increased), and age of mother at first birth (which was older and represented an "enormous difference in relative risk"). The researchers noted that if the "expected mortality rate" because of these increases was also factored in, the true decline in mortality during the decade of this study was likely closer to 20 percent, rather than the nominal 8 percent.[5] So why the decrease?

The researchers report: "For at least ten years, up until 1978, and probably for longer than that, milk and dairy products in Israel were contaminated by extraodinarily high levels of [four] pesticides:(a)-BHC (benzene hexachloride), (g)-BHC (lindane), DDE, and DDT. . . . There is evidence these high levels of pesticide contamination were bioconcentrated after entering the human food chain."[6] Mean concentration was 1,000 to 28,000 parts per billion, or five to one hundred times greater than levels observed in the United States. What these researchers discovered was that contrary to their expectations based on overall risk factors, death rates from breast cancer dropped when pesticide use was banned—and the influence was immediate and without relationship to other risk factors.

On April 21, 1993, headlines across the country proclaimed "Breast Cancer, DDT Exposure Linked in Study." Finally, even the *Journal of the National Cancer Institute* is reporting that evidence is mounting on what many have suspected for years—that is, that DDT used on our foods and the feed of animals raised for consumption is now appearing to cause a rise in breast cancer in U.S. women over fifty. Dr. Mary S. Wolff of Mt. Sinai School of Medicine in New York observed that women exposed to DDT have a four-fold risk of developing breast cancer. Significantly higher blood levels of DDE (the metabolized form of DDT) occurred in women with breast cancer. "It has been hypothesized that diets high in animal fat may therefore increase human organochlorine contamination. Over time, these compounds may trigger breast cancer by disrupting normal cell regulation processes in sensitive tissues of the breast . . . the upward shift among older women is also consistent with the historical pattern of accumulation of organochlorine residue in the environment,"[7] states Wolff. Ironically, it was Rachel Carson who began the war on DDT with her revolutionary book *Silent Spring.*[8] Carson herself became a casualty of breast cancer soon after she hypothesized in the 1960s that such chemicals have long-term effects. Now, exactly 30 years later, we are witnessing the validation of her theory.

The more informed I became, the easier it was to avoid the substances that most threatened my particular situation and ultimately my wellness. Having studied the risk factors and exposures described earlier in "Searching for the Cause," I theorized that my immune system had become overwhelmed by environmental and lifestyle challenges. What I ate and drank, all the prescription drugs I had taken, and all the environmental carcinogens to which I was exposed represented a long-term and collective bombardment that eventually made it impossible for my immune system to cope with the production of mutated cells. I didn't believe my immune system had failed me or was incapable of being restored. Instead, my cancer was an indicator that my immune system was desperately in need of a concentrated rebuilding program.

I thought of my cancer problem as being like a small airplane in flight that experiences trouble. If the engine starts to sputter, the pilot has several choices. She can stay calm and work with what she has, such as checking her fuel supply and finding a favorable place to land. Or she can focus on the sputtering, apply ear plugs, and spend time attacking the annoying sounds. The latter seems to be the current medical approach to cancer—eliminate the symptoms while praying that they don't return, without attempting to address the cause. I question whether this head-in-the-sand approach to treatment may actually threaten our ability to fully recover.

What I needed immediately was to protect and strengthen my damaged immune system, to make it my ally against the cancer and promote a new healthy environment for my cells. Changing my diet was my first line of action, along with minimizing environmental toxins and outside stress, while I continued to evaluate other treatment options (see chapter 7, "Treatment Alternatives"). I began learning about what foods I needed—and what foods I needed to avoid—to fuel the rebuilding of my system. Oriental herbs, visualization, acupuncture, and yoga provided the basis of my early program, along with a diet of no added fat, no refined sugar, and no refined flour. I immediately experienced increased energy, clearer thinking, and a more positive outlook, which reinforced my interest and desire to continue with this approach.

HEALTH PROMOTION WITH FOOD

All the food I ate was organic: free of additives, pesticides, preservatives, antibiotics, steroids, and hormones. More than ever I understood the old adage "We are what we eat." I now saw, for the first time, how this applies to cell formation. If my food was toxic and "cancer promoting" because it had been treated with pesticides, fertilizers, or added hormones, then I believed these foods would serve to compound the problem. Since my system was already in peril, I could not spare even the least deviation from my commitment to consuming only clean food and water.

Clean food is unprocessed, unadulterated food. I looked for labels that said "whole, organic, no preservatives" rather than "fresh and natural," since these latter terms are often misleading and superficial. "Fresh" and "natural" are not synonymous with healthy, because most of the fresh vegetables in the local supermarket are filled with pesticides, herbicides, chemical fertilizers, and what I call petrifiers. Processes like irradiation are used to give fresh fruits and vegetables a longer shelf life.

Our markets have all types of fruits and vegetables available all year long. These out-of-season foods must be transported long distances and are often grown using different standards than those allowed in this country. This is an extravagance that we ultimately pay for with our health.[9] Paying a premium for berries that are grown outside the United States during the winter means we run the risk of increasing our consumption of pesticides that are banned in the United States.

I used to wonder why potatoes don't sprout the same way they did when I was a kid. The reality is that we do not necessarily have a better strain of potato; rather, growers are petrifying the potato so it won't sprout, which would cause waste, which is economically undesirable. Lettuce doesn't turn brown at the salad bar or in the market because it is sprayed to prevent discoloration. Unfortunately, scientists don't fully understand what these processes do to the cells of the people who eat these foods. Economic health carries greater value than the health of people.

In the end what we get is food that looks pretty but doesn't give us the kind of fuel we need to feel and look good ourselves. The food in the American diet today is basically dead. The few things it is rich in are added fat, sodium, and additives like coloring, flavoring, fortified vitamins and minerals, and preservatives. Some food is so devoid of nutrition that the manufacturers need to fortify it to meet the standards for it to be called food.

One test I use to demonstrate to friends what I'm talking about is to take them into a natural food store and have them smell the produce. Next, we go into the supermarket and try to smell the produce. There is no smell. And along with the smell, the taste has been removed. What we are left with is pretend fruit and pretend vegetables, which require accents like salt, dressing, or sauces to give them flavor. They have no intrinsic flavor of their own. Another test is to go into a restaurant and order a vegetable dish, steamed, with nothing on it. The color is there, but often that's all. There is absolutely no taste without the chef's "secret" sauce.

And eating orangish-white tomatoes in the winter is no one's preference, yet people all over the country continue to buy this tasteless excuse for a tomato and serve it on salad. Why? Because we have not been shown how to add color to our salads with red cabbage, grated carrots, slivered red radishes, and sunflower or pumpkin seeds or raisins.

More and more seasonal fresh fruits and vegetables are available that are pesticide-free, nonirradiated, and free of chemical preservatives. Fresh food *should* spoil. As consumers we can buy smaller quantities that can be used in a short time.

As consumers, women have the power to change what is offered to us in the marketplace by becoming educated, changing the way we eat and what we buy, and demanding clean food. We should read labels, and know what is in the food we buy. If the labels have ingredients that we don't recognize, we should not assume the food is okay and buy it anyway. We need to assume that if a food product contains something that sounds unusual, it is probably a coloring, preservative, additive, or flavoring.

Women have enormous power when it comes to food purchasing. With this power comes responsibility for providing nutritious meals for ourselves as well as for our family and friends. If we won't buy certain things, the growers and distributors will grow what we do buy. If we continue to buy food that is harmful to our bodies, the growers and distributors will continue to sell these products. It's really that simple.

Nutritionists today recommend a diet that is very different from the one they recommended even just a few years ago. The U.S. Surgeon

General has stated that between 35 and 60 percent of all cancers are related to diet. There is a new emphasis on whole grains and vegetables. In April 1991, the *Journal of the National Cancer Institute* reported findings that suggested eating such foods, which are high in fiber, significantly reduced the occurrence of mammary cancer in laboratory rats. Leonard Cohen states, "It shows that the fiber itself contains substances which, when they get into the bloodstream, will inhibit the formation of a mammary tumor. What seems to be happening is that fiber by some magical means that we don't understand is creating changes in the hormone system, which protects against breast cancer."[10]

Although Cohen concluded by saying that he considered these new findings "a great surprise," I was already a believer in the value of high-fiber foods, which have been recognized by our forefathers and mothers in ethnic and native foods for centuries.[11] Cabbage and carrots, in particular, are considered to be "cancer blocking" vegetables. Lightly steaming my vegetables provided me with a vitamin-rich source of fiber. I then used the vitamin-rich liquid to prepare my soups.

In the wake of new research, a discussion has also emerged about changing the way the food groups are taught in our schools. In April 1991 a controversy began when the "basic four" food groups, originally conceived by the USDA in 1956, were redefined into a "pyramid" that included fats, oils, and sweets (recommending that they be used sparingly), and showed breads, cereals, rice, pasta, and fruits and vegetables in significantly greater proportions than before (adding more fiber to the daily diet). High-fat, high-protein foods such as dairy products, eggs, meat, poultry, and even beans were recommended in smaller quantities. This graphic triangular representation came under immediate fire by lobbyists for the meat and dairy industries and was revised.[12]

When I saw the mainstream, carefully guarded representation of what constitutes a "healthy" diet start to lean toward the kind of diet I was eating, I felt certain I was on the right track. More and more research has appeared supporting the benefits of foods that once were foreign to me but now had become part of my regular diet—tofu, shoyu (made of whole soybeans, without alcohol as a preservative), green tea, cabbage, and carrots.

A colleague of mine had called me as soon as she heard about my diagnosis and recommended the macrobiotic diet. She had had remarkable success with this grain-based diet, which she had begun only after she had undergone surgery and taken chemotherapy for a year—and then found that her breast cancer had still spread to her bones. When she was told by the doctors that there was no more they could do, she began to take control of her destiny and "with God's help" discovered the story of Dr. Anthony Sattilaro. His book, *Recalled by Life,* tells about his own near-death experience and how the macrobiotic diet reversed his advanced cancer. Dr. Sattilaro eventually died, but he gained ten more productive years of life. My colleague has been free of cancer for eight years since using the diet. Both Sattilaro and my colleague did not maintain this type of diet but instead used it, just like any other treatment, for a limited period of time. My friend continues to significantly limit her dairy and meat consumption.

After using the macrobiotic diet myself for more than three years, I decided that it has its pros and cons, like most things. I credit the diet with facilitating proper elimination. I was able to eliminate toxins, unhealthy cells, congestion, and the stresses created both by my cancer and by the environment in a reasonably short period of time—approximately six months. The reality is that it takes seven years for every cell in the body to be replaced. I consider this the benchmark of what needs to be achieved, recognizing that I am still purifying my system even today. It took many years of abuse for the cancer to take hold, and it will take a similar number of years for me to rid myself of further risk.

The most serious drawback about the macrobiotic way is that this diet requires a complete reeducation about nutritional sources, and it takes time to learn how to integrate such a diet into one's daily life. Because the diet has its roots in Japanese culture, there are many new flavors, names of foods, and new ways to think about dietary balance. Opposites are often explained as though everything in the world can be described as yin (expansive) or yang (contractive). Although I learned a great deal about food and health by eating this way, I later chose to slightly change my diet so that I didn't become unnecessarily compulsive about food.

Fats and Oils

Most people have become more aware that the fat in food can be harmful, but saying that everyone needs to be on a low-fat diet is a simplistic approach to a much more complex problem. Part of this issue is the kind

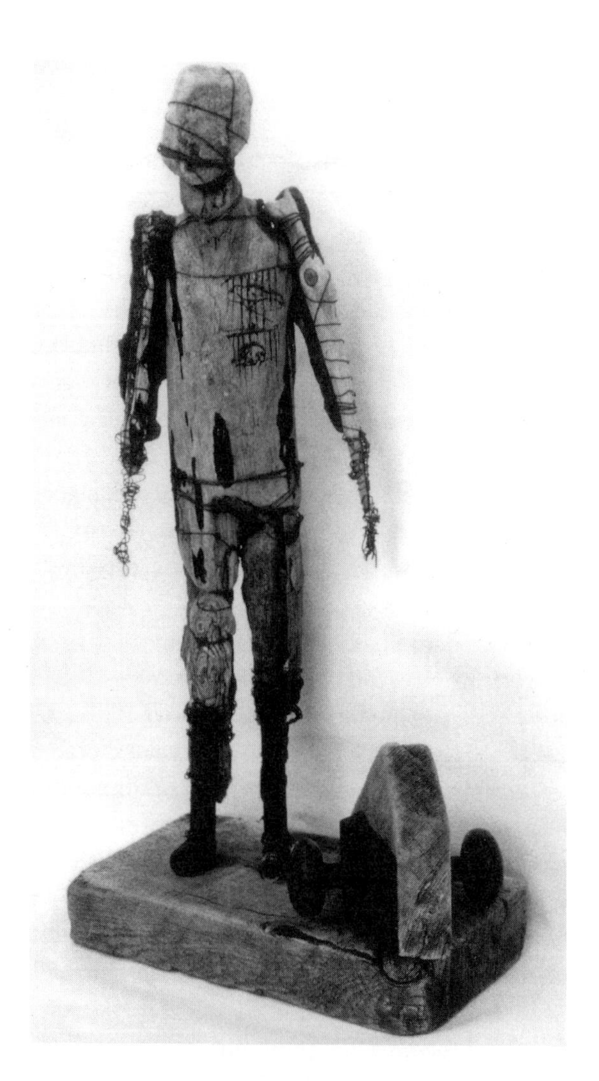

Turning East
Charlotte Franzen Ciaraldi, Vergennes, Vermont
Wood, wire, mixed media, 6½" x 12" x 25", 1992

"The headlines in the news were quoting statistics of "one in nine," so I knew I was not alone, but the numbers were frightening to hear as I began my journey. Turning East, *my second sculpture, is a reflection of my personal journey in the continuum/process of healing. It represents illumination as I travel the Medicine Wheel in all directions experiencing the past, present, and future."*

---

of fat. Animal fat, which is saturated, is the fat most harmful to our heart and arteries. It is also believed to be more harmful to women with breast cancer, since it may contain added hormones and pesticides—substances characteristically stored in fatty tissue such as breast tissue. Vegetable oils, including corn, palm, coconut, and other processed oils, constitute fats and can contribute to cancer. Mono-unsaturated fat, like olive oil, so far has not been found to be harmful.

For about eight months after my initial diagnosis, I didn't use any oil or fat other than eating fish once or twice a week and sometimes eating seeds such as sesame or sunflower. Later, I started using primarily cold-pressed organic seed oils such as sesame and sunflower oil for baking and olive oil for sautéing and for pasta sauces. Flaxseed oil is both health-building and a corrective for constipation; however, it cannot be cooked or heated and it must be refrigerated even before it is opened, because it becomes rancid if exposed to light and warm temperatures. For salads it is light and refreshing in addition to being nourishing.

Many food substitutes are coming on the market to replace fat, but these "synthetics" do not provide our bodies with the kind of fuel we need to make healthy cells. Similarly, people have been encouraged to decrease their meat intake, but chicken and dairy products are an unfortunate substitution. Chicken, now available as hormone-free and free-range, still contains saturated fat and excessive amounts of protein. The one animal product that may have cancer-blocking qualities is fish: Eskimo and Japanese women who had low rates of breast cancer ate diets high in the omega-3 fish oil found in salmon, trout, herring, and sardines.[13]

A diet high in fat and protein and low in fiber can contribute to everything from high cholesterol, clogged arteries, obesity, and heart disease to diabetes and breast cancer. A significant study conducted by Cornell University of 6,500 Chinese during 1983 and 1984 indicated that the Chinese eat 20 percent more calories than do people in America, but Americans are still 25 percent fatter. While 38 to 40 percent of the calories in the U.S. diet come from fat, only *15 percent* of the calories in the Chinese diet come from fat. Americans get 70 percent of their protein from animal foods and 30 percent from plant food. In China, 11 percent comes from animal products and 89 percent from plants. The resulting cholesterol levels are representative of the above ratios—average Western cholesterol is 212 milligrams per 100 milliliters, compared with an average of 127 milligrams in China.[14]

Foods that provide "convenience" are often the highest in fat, salt, and sugar. The flavors that Americans crave are the substances that we now know cause the greatest harm. Salt is a common preservative. Sugar is found in everything from common table salt to toothpaste. (For pure salt, I use a high-quality sea salt.) Fat is used to provide a rich flavor in everything from breads and bakery goods to snack foods.

Although at first I decided to change my diet on a provisional basis, saying to myself, "I'll give this a try for one month and see if I feel better or notice any difference," I also began to look for research to give me more incentive and validate my decision. I didn't have to look too far. The *Journal of the National Cancer Institute* reported in February 1989 (the same month that I was diagnosed) that "a positive association exists between breast cancer and consumption of dairy products, particularly those rich in fat, such as high-fat cheese and whole milk." The study recommends that women reduce their total fat to less than 30 percent of calorie intake, less than 10 percent from saturated fat, or less than 6 percent from animal proteins, as this "may be strongly protective against breast cancer."[15]

An earlier study conducted at Harvard Medical School and Brigham and Women's Hospital has demonstrated that reducing dietary fat levels to 30 percent is not enough to make a difference. The NIH is now studying reducing the levels to 20 percent.[16]

A Canadian study published in 1991 also convincingly supports the relationship betweeen dietary fat and breast cancer. The study followed 57,000 women who ate a high-fat diet and determined that the women in the study who consumed the most fat had a "35 percent greater risk of disease than those who consumed the least."[17]

Initially I decided to eliminate dairy products only because I concluded that they were filled with hormones, steroids, and antibiotic residues and were also too high in protein and fat. Later this decision helped me to identify my lactose sensitivity. Chronic skin problems, sinus problems, asthma, and allergies disappeared when I stopped consuming all dairy foods.

Like meat, dairy foods have long been associated with prosperity. My parents, after living through the Depression, felt successful when they were able to serve steak, leg of lamb, pork chops, fried chicken, and pizza on a regular basis. These foods, we were told, were "good for us."

Ice cream was always in the freezer and available for dessert or as a late-night snack. Chocolate milk, cheese sandwiches, lasagna, hamburgers, and hot dogs made up a supposed-to-be healthy lunch.

Dairy products seem to be the most difficult food for people to give up. Some people buy into the idea that if they are lactose intolerant, all they need to do is take Lactaid®. This is once again a way of removing the symptoms while ignoring the cause. Although the human being is the only mammal that continues to drink milk after weaning, most people believe unquestioningly that everyone needs milk throughout their life.

Our obsession with milk has caused the United States to do everything from undercutting family farmers because there is too much milk to funding scientists with tax dollars so that they can experiment with growth hormones. Fewer cows are now able to produce a greater volume of milk. If any product is an indicator about how food is used to leverage social conditions, it is milk.

The United States economy is driven by what could be called a "food standard" that seems to date from around 1955, when the USDA introduced the famous four food groups. When the United States government realized there would never be enough gold to back its currency, it had to find an unlimited, but cherished, substitute—like food, especially milk. Americans are now faced with health problems, such as osteoporosis,[18] generated because people have been encouraged to consume foods that contain large amounts of fat and protein.

But we do not need milk, and several doctors have published books to explain why.[19] Dr. John McDougall, for instance, explains how Bantu women in Africa have no osteoporosis, typically have ten children, and don't ever drink milk after their own early nursing.[20]

By the mid-1950s people had started to forget that those picturesque cows carry infectious diseases: typhoid in the 1800s, tuberculosis in the early 1900s, and to this day, bovine leukemia. Because of the diseases transmitted by animals through their meat and milk, as well as all the products made from milk, cows are given antibiotics and steroids. Every bite of cheese is also a serving of hormones. Additionally, cow's milk needs to be pasteurized (which also destroys enzymes in the milk that are needed by humans to digest it) to kill the viruses.

Without dairy products in my diet, however, I needed to find another natural source of calcium and vitamin D. Sea vegetables, like nori, *arame*, or kelp, and dark-green leafy vegetables like cooked kale and collards, proved to be an appealing high-fiber calcium source. I started to think of milk as the lazy man's calcium because it doesn't need to be chewed. Sunlight is our best source of vitamin D which enables our bodies to better absorb the calcium.

Watching What We Drink

After I started eating a primarily organic diet, I also took a closer look at the water I was drinking and cooking with. Living with chemicals in my water supply seems to be counterproductive to my desire to discharge the toxins in my body. City or "tap" water, which is treated with chlorine, is considered by some people to be dangerous and carcinogenic. About six weeks into my new way of eating, I began to wash my vegetables in, cook with, and drink only filtered water. Since I was working to flush the toxins from my body, I figured that my kidneys should be refreshed with a clean water source.

Breast cancer—having it or the fear of getting it—was a great motivator for changing many of my habits. I gave up caffeine as soon as the doctor confirmed that I had a suspicious lump and said that I needed to have a mammogram. She told me that it might be worth while to give up caffeine because sometimes this helps lumps to disappear. (I have since learned that all the gourmet coffee I had been enjoying is also filled with chemicals applied when it's grown and processed.) Nonetheless, Dr. Love reports in her book that early studies showing a relationship between reduced caffeine consumption and a benefit for fibrocystic disease were extrapolated to include breast cancer and were in themselves based on faulty study design. Later studies could not prove a correlation, and in fact one showed coffee drinkers to have a lower incidence of breast cancer. Finally she states, "Some women have found that reducing caffeine in their diets has helped alleviate breast symptoms. We have no medical evidence to back it up, but it works for them and you might want to try it for a while and see if it helps you."[21]

Giving up caffeine was no small task for me. My prime difficulty was deciding what to drink. It was winter, so I wanted something hot, and herbal tea never quite satisfied me the way coffee or a Tab did. My first day without caffeine was the hardest. I had a very intense headache, different from any other headache I had ever experienced—this one felt as though I had been hit by a truck. I was also very sleepy and lethargic. After about three days I got over my desire to have a "fix" and found reasonable alternatives that offered the flavor and taste of coffee. It was several weeks before I discovered grain coffee, so by then the "real" coffee taste was a more distant memory and perhaps made this an easier substitute.

The relationship between alcohol intake and breast cancer risk is still under investigation. More than 50 studies have examined this issue between 1977 and 1993 and the results have not been able to demonstrate a consistent link. Dr. Lynn Rosenberg and her colleagues conducted an extensive review of the evidence through 1992.[22] Studies have examined types of alcohol—wine, beer, and liquor—durations and quantity, as well as user charactistics — women who are pre- and post-menopausal, estrogen users, lean women, American or living in other countries. Presently no one is willing to suggest that women who are at high risk, or even those who have had breast cancer, should avoid alcohol. Nonetheless, there are some interesting findings that do suggest a relationship does exit. For example, when increased risk has been demonstrated it appeared in populations drinking as few as 1–2 drinks per week, those before age 30 and between ages 50–65, those drinking all types of alcohol, lean women, and those who are users of noncontraceptive estrogens.

The authors suggest that confounding results may be due to study design. Still, they do offer some insight on the mechanism of alcohol consumption which has been associated more directly to an elevated risk of oral, pharyngeal, laryngeal, esophageal, and liver cancers.

> Alcohol metabolism produces acetaldehyde, which is a mutagen and cocarcinogen. It has been suggested that alcohol may influence the risk of breast cancer through effects on pituitary prolactin secretion, metabolism and clearance of estrogen by the liver, or pineal melatonin production. The effects of alcohol on these factors and the roles of prolactin, estrogen, and melatonin in the etiology of breast cancer are not clearly defined.[23]

SKIN HEALTH, SUNLIGHT, AND VITAMIN D

Whenever someone talks about the cancer-producing effects of the sun, I consider how the color of my skin has lightened to a healthy pinkish tone since I eliminated toxic foods and water from my diet. I don't believe in intentionally baking or burning my skin, but I think most of the sun blocks on the market today present another set of hazards. Once I started reading food labels to assure I wasn't putting unwanted chemical additives and preservatives *into* my body, I realized that I also needed to be more sensitive to what I put *on* my body. I can't help but wonder if the reason people get skin cancer might not have more to do with body toxins accumulating at points of damaged skin tissue and perhaps have less to do with natural exposure to the sun itself.

Lotions, perfumes, makeups, soaps, and shampoos are all absorbed through the skin, just as though they were consumed. Our skin is the largest organ of the body and just as relevant to cell health. The skin is alive and breathing, releasing poisons from within and absorbing vitamin D from the sunlight.

Vitamin D is absorbed both through the eyes and through the skin. In the winter in places like the northeastern United States, it becomes critical for people to have exposure either to sunlight or to a light source such as Vitalite, a florescent bulb that simulates sunlight. Light triggers both vitamin D and vitamin A receptors, which in turn stimulate the ovaries and natural estrogen production. In 1989, a group of London doctors examined the role of vitamin D in controlling breast-cancer cell proliferation. Although vitamin D as an oral supplement proved to be a problem because of its toxicity, *in vivo* studies showed that vitamin D applied topically three times weekly produced "significant inhibition of tumor progression."[24] The objective of developing a vitamin-D treatment that would supplement chemotherapy treatments was not achieved.

There is evidence to suggest that other sources of vitamin D, such as sunlight or Vitalite, may be beneficial for recovering breast-cancer patients. Scientists are still studying this relationship, but I believe vitamin D has a direct effect on melatonin (see the section in the chapter "Searching for the Cause" for more about the relationship between melatonin, sunlight, and hormonal health).

CHEWING, DIGESTION, AND ELIMINATION

Diet does not just pertain to what we eat. How we eat, and how we metabolize, utilize, and eliminate what we eat, are equally important. Chewing has a healing benefit because it activates the digestive system and a special hormone called parotin. I always thought when my mother told me, "Chew your food," she was just trying to get me to stop talking so much at the dinner table. Now I've learned that the parotin activated by chewing provides several important immune-system benefits: it stimulates cell metabolism, destroys gastric juices, and stimulates the thymus gland, thereby producing more T-cells.[25]

Getting healthy is closely related to efficient elimination. Bowel movements are necessary at least four times per day. It was at one time considered acceptable to have one bowel movement per day, but the reality is if a person has only one bowel movement, the food that sits in the intestines ferments, and becomes harmful, and these harmful substances are reabsorbed into the body.

To achieve the best level of elimination we need to eat more vegetables and grains and to chew them thoroughly. Carbohydrates are actually digested in our mouths, not our stomachs. These food groups have nutrients that are not available in animal foods. They are also naturally low in fat and can assist us in absorbing the other food we eat. Only with regular elimination can our intestines do the job they were made to do—recycle nutrients and remove waste. Once I stopped eating flour and animal products and started eating more whole grains, my elimination process greatly improved.

If our body starts to overheat and break down (just like a car that never gets its oil changed), it's time to take a look at our diet and ease of elimination. An intestinal logjam causes us to consume enormous amounts of fluids to satisfy our thirst, lower our body temperature, and stay cool. It wasn't until I dramatically changed my diet that I realized this kind of fluid intake isn't normal or necessary when we eat properly.

As soon as I began eating a healthy diet, I also began eliminating toxins from every part of my body. I had to learn to appreciate this as a "desirable" outcome even though at times it was horrifying to see and smell what was inside of me. Sometimes I took special measures to expedite this elimination—for instance, with a garlic flush. For several days in a row, three to five depending on my condition, I would squeeze a whole bulb of organic garlic into cheesecloth, then wring out the garlic juice. Next, I combined the garlic juice with the juice of one organic lemon, two tablespoons of olive oil, and approximately four ounces of hot water.

I drank this "tea" mixture every morning before eating breakfast or consuming any other liquid. The purpose was to cleanse my liver and intestines of parasites, which improves the functioning of both organs.

The results were phenomenal. The first day was the hardest. I made sure I didn't have any appointments and worked at home alone. By day two, the garlic tea seemed sweet and pleasant to the taste. I'm told that this is an indication that it's working. A shower and brushing of the skin help to remove all the toxins and parasites that seep out through the skin, so for three years I brushed my skin every morning when I showered to assist in this elimination process (health food stores sell brushes specifically designed for the skin).

My first experience with the garlic flush occured after the house well had been contaminated and I had a definite parasitic condition from drinking this bad water for over a month. In the shower, on the morning of the second day of the garlic flush, I felt as though I had been exorcised—freed from some unexplainable possession.

My macrobiotic counselor had observed on my first visit that my kidneys were struggling to manage the toxic condition of my body. He said that the very deep, dark circles under my eyes were an indicator that my kidneys were in deep distress. The circles had become so pronounced that I once thought I looked like a raccoon. No amount of makeup would conceal this problem. I had even consulted a plastic surgeon, before I knew about my cancer, to see if he could correct this problem. Instead, he offered to remove the tiny lines around my eyes but told me that nothing could be done about the darkness because it was "hereditary." His assessment seems ludicrous to me today, since I now know that any Oriental doctor would have recognized my dark circles as an indication of my impaired kidney condition. Over the years, as I have restored my health, the dark circles have gradually improved, but they can still return like a barometer of my kidneys' sensitivity to toxins.

The presence of toxins in our bodies may be indicated by a lack of normal coloration of the skin—especially noticeable on the hands and gums—or by skin irritation such as rashes, sores, or blisters. Other indicators include frequent headaches after eating, achiness or loss of muscle strength, fatigue or listlessness, congestion in joints, allergies, chronic or progressive degenerative disease, body odor, tooth decay, and gum problems.

As I began to discharge the old toxins, I experienced what some alternative health practitioners call a "healing crisis." These occasions were marked by flu-like symptoms: fever, diarrhea, nausea, headache,

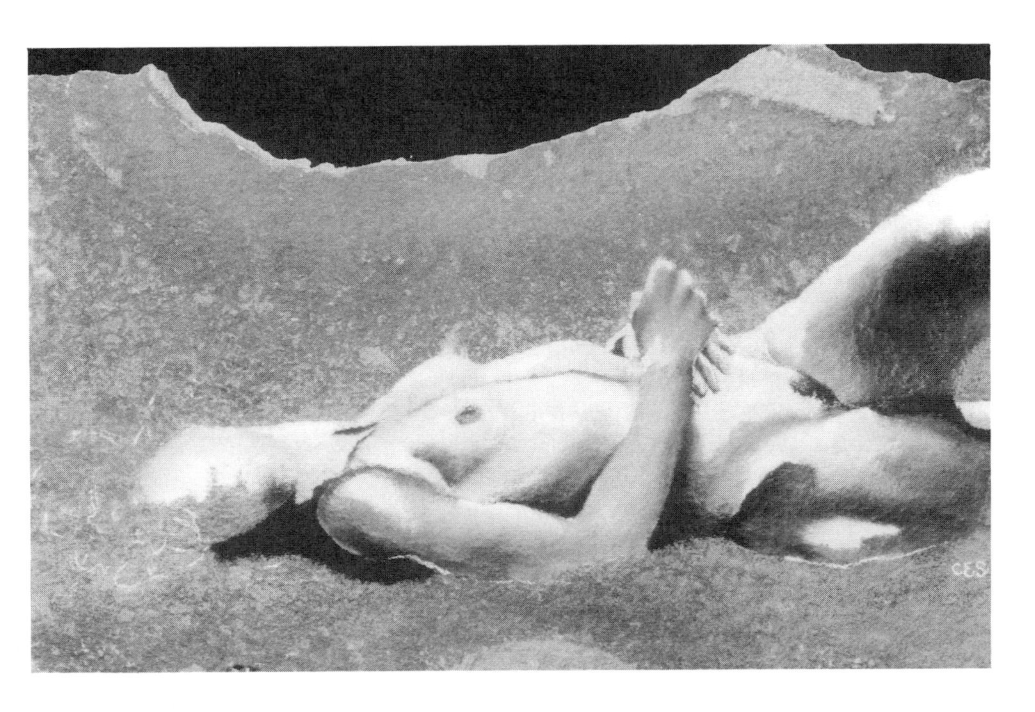

Laura No. 16
Constance Eger Shneider, Elburn, Illinois
Pastel on bluestone, 24" x 14", 1991

"My surgery and radiation treatments resulted in lack of stamina, lack of strength, and numbness in my working arm. In my garage was a flat, broken patio stone. It was just a stone and not as intimidating as paper or canvas. Being able to sit at my drawing table and work slowly on this rock gave me the confidence to begin again."

and achiness. They lasted only twenty-four hours and disappeared without any particular treatment other than adjustment of my diet. After the first few occurrences I was able to distinguish the symptoms, and instead of panicking—thinking I was getting sicker—I relaxed and acknowledged that I was getting healthier. What I learned was that toxin removal produces symptoms similar to those produced by a small amount of poison as the toxins exit. This reaction had been less obvious at the time of ingestion; when I was ingesting a multitude of health-diminishing substances I was already feeling generally numb and out of sorts and was less capable of detecting the reaction.

Through my skin, perspiration, sinuses, and bowels I continued to gradually discharge years of toxic accumulation. Now I see that when people have unpleasant body odors, bad breath, and offensive—sometimes disgusting—excrement, it's because of what is inside their bodies. I was shocked to see how polluted my own body had become over the years. I knew that what I was doing was working because the pinkish color began to return to my skin.

As women, even when we exercise we don't perspire as much and eliminate these toxins at the same rate men do. When I go to the gym for sports-fitness class, I'm both grossed-out and impressed by how much the men sweat, while women doing the same workout have only a slight amount of perspiration. This makes it even more necessary for women to be cognizant of what we eat. Now I think of a diet not as a way to lose weight but rather as a way to clean house. Weight loss is just one of the many beneficial side effects that come with this kind of health-restoring program. Weight loss was one way for me to eliminate unhealthy cells and excess estrogen. Healthy eating has meant higher energy for me, because my body doesn't have to work so hard to digest and excrete the excess garbage hidden in the average American's diet.

GETTING STARTED

Like housecleaning, healthy eating isn't something we can do once and not worry about again. It is one of those activities that needs to become routine—a part of our lives. Having a mental picture of how some of my cells had been created from hamburgers, pork chops, cottage cheese, and chocolate-chip cookies made it much easier for me to stick with my dietary changes.

Cleaning out my cabinets and refrigerator helped me to get a fresh start. Every cereal box, cookie, and piece of cheese was removed—even the old spices. Gradually I began to replace my old standbys with new canisters of whole grains (brown rice, oats, wheat berries, quinoa, teff, millet), beans (lentils, black soy beans, adzuki, garbanzo), and sea vegetables. Cornstarch, which is highly processed, was replaced with a Japanese root called *kuzu*.

Kuzu has many wonderful healing properties. To make a tea that relieves stomach disorders, bloating, and diarrhea, as well as general achiness or muscle pain, dissolve one tablespoon *kuzu* root in eight ounces of cold water. Grate fresh ginger to equal one teaspoon, and squeeze it in your hand to release the juice into the *kuzu* water. Warm the mixture over low heat, stirring regularly to prevent lumpiness. When the liquid becomes clear and filmy, add up to half a teaspoon *tamai shoyu* and drink as a beverage. This tea can be used as often as necessary to relieve symptoms. *Kuzu* with *umeboshi* paste relieves sore throats and cold symptoms.

White sugar and honey were also removed. Refined sweeteners—including honey—are burned quickly and give the body false indicators of highs and lows. Sweeteners that are more slowly released into energy include rice syrup, barley malt, and *mirim*. On special occasions maple syrup can also be used.

Products like white flour, refined sugar, and white rice are incomplete carbohydrates. They can be stored in our tissue as fat since they do not contain all the necessary parts—such as the germ and the bran—to be fully metabolized. Some people use carbohydrates more efficiently than others. Generally, our metabolism and level of exercise will influence how we process carbohydrates. Complete carbohydrates help our bodies stay warm in colder climates. It is indeed unfortunate that this "essential" food group was practically eliminated from the American diet as refining became popular and societally coveted.

For me it wasn't enough to eat a particular way just because someone told me to do it. I wanted to know how it worked and why, so I kept reading and looking at other literature. I learned to adjust what I ate as my body required. There is no one way to eat. No one food is suitable every morning for breakfast. In the beginning of my healing, I needed miso soup for breakfast with whole grains, rice, oats, or millet porridge.

Later I added whole-grain cold cereal with rice milk for the summer, and rolled oats in the winter. I changed what I ate with the seasons and ate what made me feel better. Sometimes that might even be a whole-grain muffin or a piece of whole-wheat toast, but it never was a doughnut or coffee cake. Other times it was cooked kale or raw carrots. Just because it was breakfast time didn't mean I couldn't have soup, salad, or vegetables. Fortunately, there are no "refrigerator police" to enforce when we eat our vegetables. At first it felt a bit weird not eating the kinds of breakfast foods I had been raised on. Now I just listen to my body and eat what works for me, and I don't worry about being weird.

The most important thing I learned from simplifying my diet is how my body responds to different kinds of food. Sometimes I can't eat any flour products; at other times, as when I'm doing a lot of exercise, grains cause me too much lactic acid. The healthier I became the more I was able to broaden my diet. Nonetheless my goal is not to someday eat ice cream or chocolate again. To me these foods are like drugs—too dangerous to experiment with. I "just say no" permanently and find healthy alternatives like frozen Rice Dream and tofu brownies!

The crucial aspect of a workable, healthy diet is having a full range of food types rather than all fruit or all raw foods. I also learned that the foods need to be suitable to where you live and what is physically possible for you to prepare or have prepared. I did not ever try to weigh one regimen against another. Instead, I adopted and adapted the macrobiotic diet so that it became a lifestyle change rather than a diet. I still eat very selectively and often travel with my own food. (At the end of this chapter I have included a self-discovery questionnaire and weekly log.)

I also believe foods containing sugar and caffeine actually cause an altered state of consciousness. They cause us to crave more, to feel giddy, and maybe even to obsess with how much is enough. They have no nutritional value whatsoever.

I feel a sense of freedom now that I am not controlled by fat or sugar cravings. Sometimes, though it's hard for me to believe, the smell of fresh buttered popcorn or rich ice cream actually turns my stomach. Having my diet under control helps me be more responsible for what I put into my body. Understanding how food affects the health of my cells helps me make educated food choices in all situations.

More people are starting to realize that we are killing ourselves with what we eat—more than with any other factor including tobacco. (It really doesn't take a surgeon general's report to see the seriousness of this problem. Just take a look at the people at your local supermarket— 25 percent of all Americans are overweight, and many have some related physical limitation because of this condition.) When I began to examine diet research, I was glad to see how many doctors and health-conscious people are now publishing books about the relationship of diet to health. In my bibliography I have included the names of the books I found to be most helpful.

MINIMIZING ENVIRONMENTAL DAMAGE TO HEALTH

The kinds and extent of change I needed to make in my external environment, and for how long, depended on how much reserve I had left in my battered immune system. As my immune system began to rebuild I noticed that I became less sensitive to several environmental substances that I had initially identified as my "enemies."

I was hypersensitive to electromagnetic energy during the initial phase of my healing. My computer was off-limits for several months; it wouldn't even boot up if I stood closer than eight feet. I permanently removed the electric blanket from my bed when I learned that it interfered with fetal development in pregnant women and had been traced to childhood cancers. If I was going to produce new healthy cells, I had to take all the same precautions that an expectant mother would. I treated my own body as though it were giving birth to a new life—*my* new life. I avoided air travel because of the ambient radiation, and I avoided swordfish, which is high in mercury; both of these things are considered a threat to a developing fetus.

MINIMIZING STRESS

Emotional reactions can suppress or stimulate disease-fighting white blood cells and trigger the release of adrenal-gland hormones and neurotransmitters. Virtually every illness can be influenced, positively or negatively, by a person's mental state.[26]

It seemed as though the stress caused by the diagnosis was enough to send my fragile immune system over the edge. I felt depressed and unmotivated to do anything, even eat. My body felt almost too heavy to move around. Fortunately, my new diet became a source of energy rather than of additional stress, as I would have expected.

My immune system also seemed to be more vulnerable to other potentially weakening events. Drug or radiation treatments or surgery would become additional stresses to this system. Personal crises—with relationships, finances, or personal property—can add more stress and more vulnerability to an already faltering system. Although these were impossible events to control, there were times when I needed to back off any type of intensive routine and spend additional time resting, meditating, and taking care of myself.

CONCLUSION

Initially, few of the doctors I consulted were willing to admit that breast cancer is a chronic disease. Many held out the hope that if I would just submit to their prescribed treatments, then, more likely than not, I would be fine.

Their treatments involved adding more harmful, carcinogenic substances to my body. What I decided to do was only what was best for me, not necessarily what I think would be best for all women. The shock of the treatment process can become so encompassing that some women become unable to get their immune systems to rally back to recovery. Since no one could tell me why some immune systems rally and others default, I felt that taking the standard therapy was a huge gamble. I simply could not subject my body to such an assault.

Having seen some friends try diet and alternative treatments as a last resort rather than for restorative reasons, my own opinion is that it's probably a little easier to boost the immune system before chemotherapy and radiation add to the body's toxic condition. Nonetheless, I have also seen people who have undergone all the treatments and for whom a subsequent dietary change has proved to be very useful. As my macrobiotic counselor said during my first visit, "What do you have to lose? Whatever treatment you choose, a healthier diet will support you."

Yet there are still doctors today who tell their patients that diet doesn't make a difference and who are taking away an individual's desire to do more than take her medicine. Doctors I consulted about chemotherapy tried to reassure me that the earlier the cancer is caught, the healthier the immune system, and that because I was healthy and strong my body would "spring right back." They offered this metaphor to convince me that someone in my condition had little to worry about. On the other hand, a woman with more advanced disease is told she should participate in clinical trials because there is no alternative. Neither justification provides any real medical basis for attacking our own body with poisons. Ultimately, we can only do what we believe in, because if we believe in it—whatever the treatment—it will have a better chance of succeeding.

I realized that even "nice" doctors give high-dose therapeutic radiation and chemotherapy because they believe they are offering the best service. It took me a long time to understand that just because they are *nice people,* and just because they believe in these treatments, doesn't make their treatments the only or the best solution.

Many people would rather take a pill to lower their cholesterol, prevent pregnancy, or stop a headache than stop and take inventory of the alternatives. The world isn't really so dualistic that everything must be polarized into one route or another, good or bad, right or wrong. Yet often our choices are reduced to this kind of dualistic thinking. It is as though our only option for survival is take the treatment or die. What about the women who take the treatment and still die? Or more to the point, what about the women who don't take the treatment and live?

Let's allow ourselves to consider the miracle of our body's immune system and how it goes into action to save us from perishing. The immune system wants to support us, but we must return this support in every way we can. The immune system may be the closest link we have to our souls. Our immune systems give us lots of time to experiment, try things out, even exert outright abuse. Like an old workhorse, the immune system kicks in and helps us to recover. When cancer germinates in our cells, however, the medical community responds by attacking our single greatest defense. Even though some doctors might argue that this is a byproduct of the treatment, I see the immune system as being largely ignored by medicine today.

An oncologist remarked to me one day when I went in for a checkup that because of AIDS there is finally money available to research the immune system. "Up until now," she said, "no one even looked at how the immune system worked." I was startled at her offhandedness toward the threat of AIDS, but at the same time I felt that what she was saying probably had some validity. Cancer treatments in use today were designed before scientists fully understood the role of the immune system. Chemotherapy and radiation are, I believe, like a twentieth-century dinosaur that is destined to become extinct.

EATING HABITS ASSESSMENT

My goals for changing the way I eat are:

____

____

____

Circumstances in which I have the most difficulty controlling my eating (circle all that are appropriate):

	Mindful alternatives to my habitual response
When I'm really hungry	________________
Right after I've gone food shopping	________________
When I'm preparing a meal	________________
When I'm clearing the table	________________
At parties, holidays, or vacations	________________
If certain people offer me food	________________
After an emotional upset	________________
At certain times of the day	________________
When I smell food cooking	________________
When I watch television	________________
Before going to bed	________________
If I'm around others who are eating	________________
When I come home from work	________________

The foods that I crave the most are

Sweet	Sour	Cold	Hard
Spicy	Salty	Crunchy	Chewy

I usually eat (circle any that apply):

Alone	With family or friends
Three regular meals	Continuously graze—5 to 6 small meals
Small portions	A plateful to feel that I got my share
Fast or on the run	In a relaxed manner
Dessert	Salty snacks

TIPS FOR EATING MANAGEMENT

1. **Shopping:** Don't shop when you're hungry. Prepare a shopping list and don't buy anything that's not on your list. Try to shop at off-peak times so that the experience is less stressful. Shop with a friend; make it a social time, not a chore. If you're stuck in line, occupy your mind, notice the other shoppers, read a magazine, or start writing your check.
2. **Storing Food:** Put tempting snacks in cupboards. Keep fresh vegetables on shelves where you won't forget them. Opaque containers may cause you to forget about foods; use clear glass containers for storage.
3. **Meal Preparation:** Resist the temptation to eat food scraps when chopping. Save these small pieces in a special container for soups. Ask for help. Just having another person wash vegetables, or do some grating or peeling, makes a huge difference. Do preparation in small amounts. Wash all the vegetables to be used in the meal, then take a break. Start the rice, then go make some phone calls or set the table. Chop vegetables only when you are going to use them to get maximum nutrient value.

   Preparation sequence can make a difference in how long things take. Start the longest-cooking items first. This may be the rice or beans. Better yet, prepare beans in advance. Next make the dessert; this allows for baking or setting time. Make the soup, vegetables, fish, and salads last. Salad ingredients can be washed and chilled hours before the meal for the best results. The dressing can also be prepared in advance. Think through the meal in advance. Write down starting times when preparing for guests or complex menus.
4. **Mealtime Eating:** Variety is the key to meal enjoyment. Meals should be colorful and have varying textures, distinctive flavors, and new ingredients. Take your time to savor the flavors. Never eat standing up; this can impair digestion. Enjoy seconds of soups, vegetables, and grains if you don't feel satisfied. Grains are the most filling of the foods. Chew your food thoroughly before swallowing. Remember, carbohydrates, grains, breads, and corn are digested in your mouth, not your stomach.
5. **Clean-up:** Leftovers can be completely transformed into another meal. Small amounts of vegetables, tofu, or fish become pizza

toppings or parts of a salad or pasta dish, used in a miso broth for a quick pick-me-up, or can be marinated as an appetizer.

When you eat better, you feel better, and doing so is a way of loving ourselves.

HOW TO USE TABLE 4

The purpose of this chart is to increase your awareness about the relationship between what you eat, how you feel, and how your body responds to certain foods.

1. Copy Table 4 on the next page to help you begin a conscious eating program.
2. Note what you eat in the boxes for each meal and check off the corresponding food group below the corresponding day.
3. Observe and record how your body responds to the foods you have eaten in the response diary section of the table. Use the categories provided next to the sample table below.

	Sunday
Breakfast	miso soup w. kombu hot oats tea (Banchu)
Lunch	tempeh w. rice mushrooms steamed squash/kale
Dinner	salmon, red potatoes broccoli, mushroom sauce water, whole grain bread
Snack	raw carrots hummus rice crackers
Whole Grains	☒ ☒ ☒ ☒
Vegetables*	☒ ☒ ☒ ☒
Beans	☒ ☒ ☐ ☐
Fish	☒
Fruit	☐ ☐
Beverages	☒ ☒ ☐ ☐ ☐
*sea or land	
Response Diary	mood: up vitality: average temp: average cycle: regular skin: smooth mucus: none; gas: none elimination: regular nails: strong

Mood:	Up	Even	Down
Vitality:	Low	Average	High
Body Temperature:	Cold	Average	Hot
Menstrual Cycle:	Regular	Cramps	Heavy
Skin Textue:	Dry	Smooth	Oily
Mucus:	Nose	Eyes	Chest
Gas (after):	Breakfast	Lunch	Dinner
Elimination:	Difficult	Regular	Soft
Nails:	Brittle	Soft	Strong

	Sunday	Monday	Tuesday	Wednesday	Thursday	Friday	Saturday
Breakfast							
Lunch							
Dinner							
Snack							
Whole Grains	☐☐☐☐	☐☐☐☐	☐☐☐☐	☐☐☐☐	☐☐☐☐	☐☐☐☐	☐☐☐☐
Vegetables*	☐☐☐☐	☐☐☐☐	☐☐☐☐	☐☐☐☐	☐☐☐☐	☐☐☐☐	☐☐☐☐
Beans	☐☐☐☐	☐☐☐☐	☐☐☐☐	☐☐☐☐	☐☐☐☐	☐☐☐☐	☐☐☐☐
Fish	☐	☐	☐	☐	☐	☐	☐
Fruit	☐☐	☐☐	☐☐	☐☐	☐☐	☐☐	☐☐
Beverages	☐☐☐☐☐	☐☐☐☐☐	☐☐☐☐☐	☐☐☐☐☐	☐☐☐☐☐	☐☐☐☐☐	☐☐☐☐☐
*sea or land							
Response Diary							

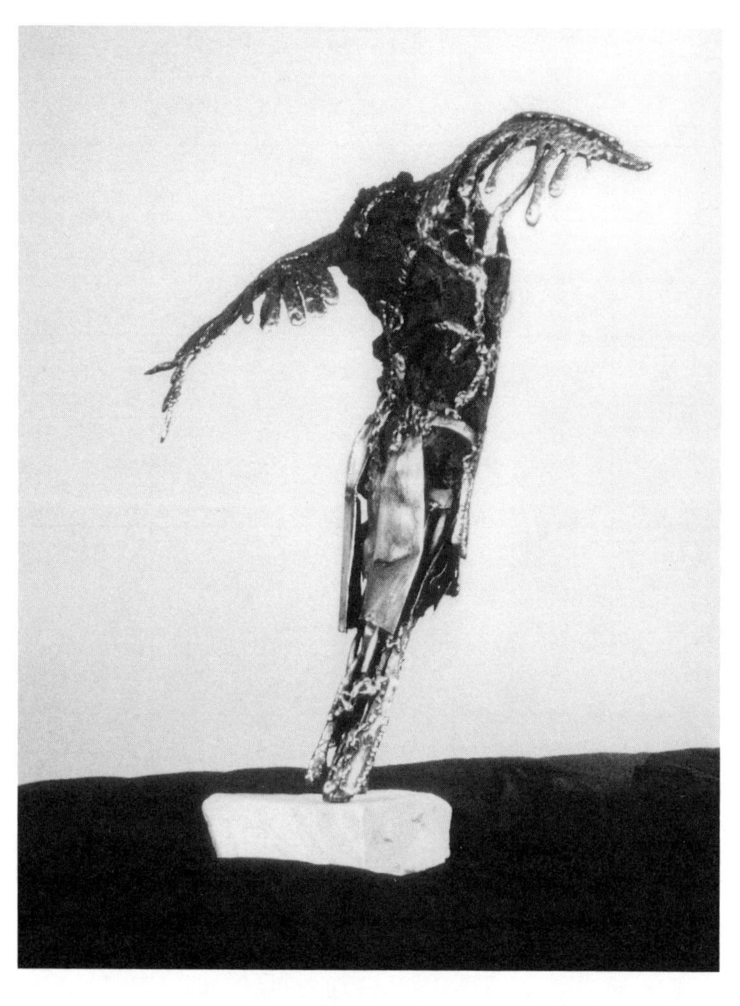

Nike of Mastectomy
Kay Minto, Susanville, California
Lava rock and aluminum, 29" x 28" x 14", 1992

"I told the surgeon that artists are given license to put the finger in the wound. It's often exceedingly painful but frequently results in a physical manifestation that not only gives us greater insight but allows us to fully experience the situation and share that experience with others in a tangible form."

6

Choosing Surgery

> *When your strategy is deep and far-reaching, then what you gain by your calculations is much, so you can win before you even fight. When your strategic thinking is shallow and nearsighted, then what you gain by your calculations is little, so you lose before you do battle. Much strategy prevails over little strategy, so those with no strategy cannot but be defeated. Therefore it is said that victorious warriors win first and then go to war, while defeated warriors go to war first and then seek to win.*
>
> Zhag Yu, *The Art of War*

Breast surgery is a serious proposition, one that I spent more than two years contemplating. My first choice was to save my breast. Initially I didn't believe my cancer represented a life-or-death situation. I wanted to remain whole. My efforts to restore my immune system had been successful to a great extent; however, this alone did not prevent the tumor from returning at the site of the original biopsy. But before I discuss my recurrence, I would like to reflect on the whole surgical process from the beginning.

I do not recommend that anyone else wait two years to have surgery. In fact, as I have said earlier, if I had known at the outset what I know today, I would have done things differently. When my cancer was first diagnosed and the biopsy was not properly executed, I needed to have additional surgery but could not find a doctor who would do the surgery I wanted. I asked for a careful excision of the area, one that would cause little or no deformity. Considering that my tumor was only the size of a pea, this did not seem like an unreasonable request. But the surgeons I saw—two men and two women—felt obligated to perform a mastectomy. One of the women offered to perform a lumpectomy, but only if I would agree to undertake radiation and possibly chemotherapy in advance of the surgery.

These options didn't fit with my early goals to not compromise my immune system and to find a less mutilating procedure than a mastectomy. I didn't feel I had a real choice about my treatment, and I was frustrated that my early-detected cancer still required a mastectomy. I felt betrayed because I had heard so much about lumpectomies and the virtues of "catching it early." This frustration motivated my search for immune-system strengthening approaches. Once I decided that surgery was mandatory, I also found the determination I needed to find the kind of surgeon who understood and respected my concerns.

In hindsight, I probably should have continued to search for a surgeon during the first six months to a year. It didn't really matter whether I saw a hundred doctors. My improved diet bought me time, and time helped me become psychologically prepared for losing my breasts if that was what was required to keep me alive. The important lesson I learned was to recognize the seriousness of breast cancer, the likelihood of a recurrence, and the need to incorporate immune-system–building treatments as an essential part of restoring health.

The medical professionals I encountered did not support my treatment of choice; instead, they confined themselves to standard medical procedures and the protection of their careers. I couldn't win by either compromising my wishes or standing by my convictions. I had to find a way to do what needed to be done and also have that be my choice. Unfortunately it took me more than two years to move beyond my frustration, my feelings of abandonment by the medical profession, and my realization that my choice wasn't really a choice at all.

Many books are available that describe surgery options and what you can expect to happen from start to finish. What isn't provided in these books is a first-person discussion of the many facets of the experience that some women don't consider until well after surgery. I would like you to have the benefit of what I learned, starting with the biopsy procedure.

THE BIOPSY

Microcalcifications that appeared on my mammogram were an indicator that cancer might exist. If I had known about this increased likelihood of a malignancy, I would have selected my biopsy surgeon more thoughtfully. Unfortunately, I did not see the mammogram or have anyone explain the findings until after the biopsy. I recommend that every woman ask to see her mammogram and be informed of the significance of its findings before she has any surgery. No biopsy is really routine. Take time to select a surgeon whom you respect and in whom you have confidence. This is an important procedure and can make a difference later on.

In my case, I felt that the biopsy procedure was minimized. The gynecological nurse practioner I had initially seen informed me by phone of the findings, and she recommended that I see the first surgeon available. When I met with this man, he reassured me by saying there was only a 15 percent chance that the tumor was malignant. The truth is this: mammography is such an imperfect method of detection that 85 percent of the biopsies performed are unnecessary; hence, only 15 percent are malignant. Of course, that did not mean that *my* chances of a negative biopsy were 85 percent; rather, of *all* women who undergo biopsy, only 15 percent prove positive. This doctor also told me, "It will be like having a mole removed." This may have reduced my anxiety, but at the same time it limited my ability to make a truly informed decision.

Having a mole removed is a procedure I have had many times, and I can assure you my biopsy procedure did not resemble it in any manner—except in the method of anesthesia, which I had reservations about.

For most people local anesthesia is completely adequate; however, I do not respond to this type of anesthesia. Although I informed the surgeon, he assured me he could properly anesthetize me. This proved not to be the case, and the nurses literally had to hold me down so the doctor could complete the biopsy procedure, which involved digging deep into my breast. This first procedure was not successful in getting clear margins, which meant the doctor had cut into the tumor and spilled cancer cells into the neighboring tissue. Although a needle with a hook at the end is inserted into the tumor so that the surgeon can locate its center, the surgeon is essentially operating blind, guesstimating how much tissue to take. Breast cancer surgeons only know for sure if they have gotten "enough" tissue *after* the pathologist has taken a look at it under the microscope and passed judgment. It it unfortunate that more doctors are not blazing new trails to refine these procedures.

Today another procedure, called stereotactic biopsy, is available at most large hospitals. It is performed in an X-ray lab and does not require a surgeon. A tissue sample of the tumor is taken with a needle for diagnostic purposes only; the procedure is quick and relatively noninvasive, and there is no attempt to obtain clear margins. The noninvasive aspect of a stereotactic biopsy makes it much more desirable than other biopsy procedures for the woman who has a benign condition. For the woman with a malignancy, it provides time to assess options before proceeding to the next step.

Preliminary pathology examinations were once routinely done during surgery. While the patient was still under general anesthesia, a sample was frozen for a quick determination of malignancy, allowing the doctor to make the decision to remove the whole breast if malignancy was confirmed. Today, more and more hospitals refuse to give out the results of the frozen section, because more detailed pathology tests might reveal conflicting outcomes. Complete pathology tests can take two to three days to produce final results. Waiting for the pathology results can be very anxiety producing, but it's better than getting a false answer.

I can't help but wonder how many women during the 1940s through the 1970s had their breasts needlessly removed on the basis of the frozen-section results, before anyone knew that this alone is a fallible method for determining malignancy.

This now mostly outdated surgical approach was known as the one-step mastectomy. Women today owe a debt of gratitude to women like Rosamond Campion, who in 1971 refused to go along with the routine one-step procedure by refusing to sign the consent form. In Campion's case, the tumor proved to be noninvasive and very small, so she was also one of the first women to ask for a lumpectomy. Rosamond remarked five years after her "pioneering" approach, "The choice I made was right for me. I do not, and cannot recommend it for every woman."[1]

An even more well-known pioneer of the two-step procedure, Rose Kushner, demanded this option for herself in 1974, when she learned that it was being used in Europe. Before then it was standard practice for a woman to go into surgery giving her doctor carte blanche to make the breast-removal decision, based on the results of the frozen section.

Twenty years later, it seems, women are still a long way from participating in truly informed consent. Although there are informed-consent laws in most states and seven states mandate full disclosure about treatment options for breast cancer, some researchers report that 80 percent of patients are not told their options.

The main problem with the two-step procedure is that most women are in such a state of shock on hearing they have breast cancer that they practically become deaf. The almost knee-jerk reaction is to do whatever the doctor recommends—and to do it fast. I hear over and over again of women who become so terrified at the thought of cancer growing in their bodies that all they can think of is getting it out. Many women forgo even a second opinion, feeling that they do not want to do anything to delay the removal by even a few days.

When I learned of my malignancy, I also learned that my insurance company required a second opinion and considered this type of surgery a nonemergency. Clearly there was a contradiction here.

Seeking out a woman surgeon for my second opinion, I was told that at this point my tumor had probably been growing for six to eight years and I had a few months before anything would change, despite the fact that the other doctor did not get clear margins. This understanding of the rate of growth is based on the doubling time of a cancerous cell.[2]

Realizing that my cancer had not occurred overnight, I became less frantic about my own situation. I reasoned that the main difference between my condition before the diagnosis and after it was a psychological difference created by the impact of being told I had breast cancer. This information alone helped me take the time I needed to make an informed decision and learn more about my surgical options.

New research has raised the question of whether there may be an optimal time of the month for premenopausal women to have breast surgery, including biopsy. Unfortunately, the data are contradictory, leaving both doctors and patients without any applicable information as to the "best" time to perform surgery.

An article originally published in the *Lancet* in May 1991 stated that premenopausal women who had operations for breast cancer during days three to twelve of their menstrual cycle had greater recurrence rates than women who had operations at other times.[3] In the ensuing months these data were disputed at five medical centers where the records of 971 patients were reviewed. Later studies, despite some similar findings, did not identify a single window in the menstrual cycle that is more favorable to the operation.

The logic of this investigation is easy to follow. If breast cancer is estrogen dependent, and a woman's menstrual cycle causes variations in the level of estrogen in her body, then perhaps there is a phase of the menstrual cycle when the tumor is less active or the condition of the breast tissue is more receptive to surgical intervention. Furthermore, women who are premenopausal seem to have more aggressive cancers and poorer survival rates; hence, one factor that might improve survival is the timing of the surgery. We are no closer to understanding the influence of menstruation on survival or recurrence than we were one hundred years ago, but studies like the one I have cited from the *Lancet* raise hope that some researchers are willing to risk controversy and perhaps even embarrassment for attempting to unravel the mysteries of the menstrual cycle and its influence on breast cancer.

TAKING TIME TO ADJUST TO THE CANCER DIAGNOSIS

Doctors sometimes contend that the shock of hearing the diagnosis can result in denial and consequent delay in getting the needed treatment. My desire to get a second opinion and to learn more about breast cancer was met with a great deal of resistance from my physicians. My decision to build up my immune system led the doctors to think that I was either in denial about the seriousness of my disease or paralyzed by the fear of the disease and surgery. Both these observations were incorrect.

I had lived with a physical limitation—strabismus—and I had recently undergone elective eye surgery to correct my crossed eyes, so I was not dismissing surgery because of fear. And I had burned my leg when I was fourteen years old; the burn had been misdiagnosed as second degree, when in reality it was a third-degree burn that required a skin graft. Since I had never received the necessary graft, people looked at my leg and asked, "What happened?"; children at the beach would point at my leg saying "Mommy, Mommy, look at her." So I already knew what it was like to live with the consequences of having a physical deformity. These experiences had a dramatic impact on my understanding of both medical miracles and the limitations of doctors. But my surgeon only knew me from what I told him and what he saw. He hadn't known me before the lump developed. He didn't know anything about my history or my desire to make an informed decision about something that would permanently change my life.

Although I had had experience with my mother's colon-cancer treatment, I was ignorant about breast cancer. All I could do was withhold consent until I could make a truly informed decision. I suppose I was also fortunate to have a slow-growing cancer that allowed me time to become educated and adjust mentally to what was for me inevitable—a mastectomy.

Since I don't subscribe to the theory that early, aggressive treatment is always better—meaning more life preserving or resulting in a "cure" (which does not exist for breast cancer)—I instead approached my breast-cancer treatment with a researched and vigilant plan of action that took me time to develop. Although waiting two and a half years before submitting to surgery may seem to some to have been risky, foolish, or outright stupid, my delay in seeking further surgical treatment is not unique. Such a delay can and does occur with breast cancer patients for a variety of reasons.

Dr. Patricia Bredenberg designed her dissertation project to examine the social-support network for women with breast cancer.[4] Her study shows that when treatment is delayed, 80 percent of the time the delay is due to physicians, not patients. Physicians might advise watching the lump, delay further diagnostic procedures because the patient is "too young," or misclassify the mass as a cyst. These conclusions are frequently arrived at without benefit of mammography, sonography, or attempted aspirations, but they can also result from false readings and false expectations of today's technology.

At the opposite extreme is the instance of a woman whom Bredenberg identifies as Carol. Carol found a lump and went to her doctor the next day. The doctor ordered a mammogram and then asked her to see a surgeon on the same day. The surgeon determined that the lump was "probably malignant," so he sent her on to an oncologist. Carol saw all the specialists within a thirty-six-hour period.

Bredenberg contends that Carol was not given the opportunity to protect herself, to prepare herself emotionally to handle this new reality. These doctors were up front about the seriousness of Carol's problem. Both Carol and her husband felt "helpless and hopeless." The result was tragic; Carol died nine months later. Whether her death was due to the aggressiveness of her cancer or to her mental state we can never know for certain. What is known from other studies and published literature is that patients who have a helpless or hopeless attitude about their diagnosis have worse survival rates.

Giving information in a caring way, educating patients at the rate they can handle it, and obtaining legal consent: each service has a distinct and different purpose. Bredenberg describes *care* as "expressions of caring, affirmation, valuing listening, accepting." The legal definition of informed consent is a good one; however, it's better in theory than in practice. Although a doctor's work appears to be highly standardized, every patient is an individual, and therefore treatment cannot always follow the same course. This ultimately leaves the *informed* part in the hands of the doctor and the *consent* part up to the terrified patient.

I wanted to have a basis for deciding on a surgical procedure, surgeon, and follow-up procedure. I wanted to retain my rights to these decisions without being abandoned by the doctors because of my questioning and delay. Both these requests, seemingly straightforward on the surface, proved to be significant challenges.

Bredenberg states, "Many studies show that information dispels uncertainty and lowers anxiety. . . . Patients value a physician's interpersonal skills more than they value his/her technical or medical competence, [however] most women felt they got neither."[5] This was also my experience. Most doctors did not welcome my questions, my desire to know, or the information I had gathered. My desire to understand fully what was to happen was often met with resistance and avoidance. This in itself became an obstacle that I had to overcome. I had to find the kind of doctor who was not threatened by a noncompliant patient. I had to find a surgeon who did not superimpose his or her own prejudices about treatment on me.

Since many surgeons are men, research provided by Bredenberg might provide insight into the feelings of the men who treat women with breast cancer. One 1982 survey demonstrated that "men regarded mastectomy as the most prominent feature of breast cancer, and felt a woman's concerns would be primarily 'cosmetic' and emotional." Although 69 percent of the male surgeons surveyed stated that a "mastectomy was the worst thing that could happen to a woman," only 28 percent of the female surgeons interviewed agreed.[6] This is not to say that females are more in tune with their patients' feelings; rather it is to say that all people have some preconceptions about this disease. These preconceptions need to be considered by the patient when she hears the doctor's opinion. It is only natural for surgeons to have a long list of experiences to base their own recommendations on.

SELECTING A SURGEON

I discovered while interviewing surgeons that this process was also my opportunity to become educated about the advantages and disadvantages of each surgical procedure. My surgeon needed to be skilled in the operating room and had to be someone with whom I was personally comfortable. I looked for someone who would answer all my questions without treating me as though I were taking too much time. The way the surgeon reacted to my questions, fears, and concerns was a good indicator of how he or she might handle my desire to be involved in my treatment decisions.

My choice of a surgeon would ultimately affect my physical appearance and my survival. The time I took to find the right surgeon gave me the edge I needed to go into surgery emotionally and physically equipped to handle the result. I learned from Lawrence LeShan's and Bernie Siegel's work that my attitude could have a direct effect on my immune system. A beneficial attitude was not something I could fabricate; I had to find resolution to my questions and be resolute about my decision.

No two doctors treat breast tumors in the same manner. I learned there is little agreement on what will produce the best results. Depending on what part of the country you live in, what doctors you see, and what protocols are being studied at the hospitals you visit and when, you will hear different recommendations.

I wanted to know more about the surgeon. I wanted to know whether he or she would perform magic or injury. Other women might tell me someone was a good surgeon, but I didn't know what their own standards were. This wasn't like going to a restaurant or a movie. The word *good* hardly seemed an adequate recommendation for what was about to take place.

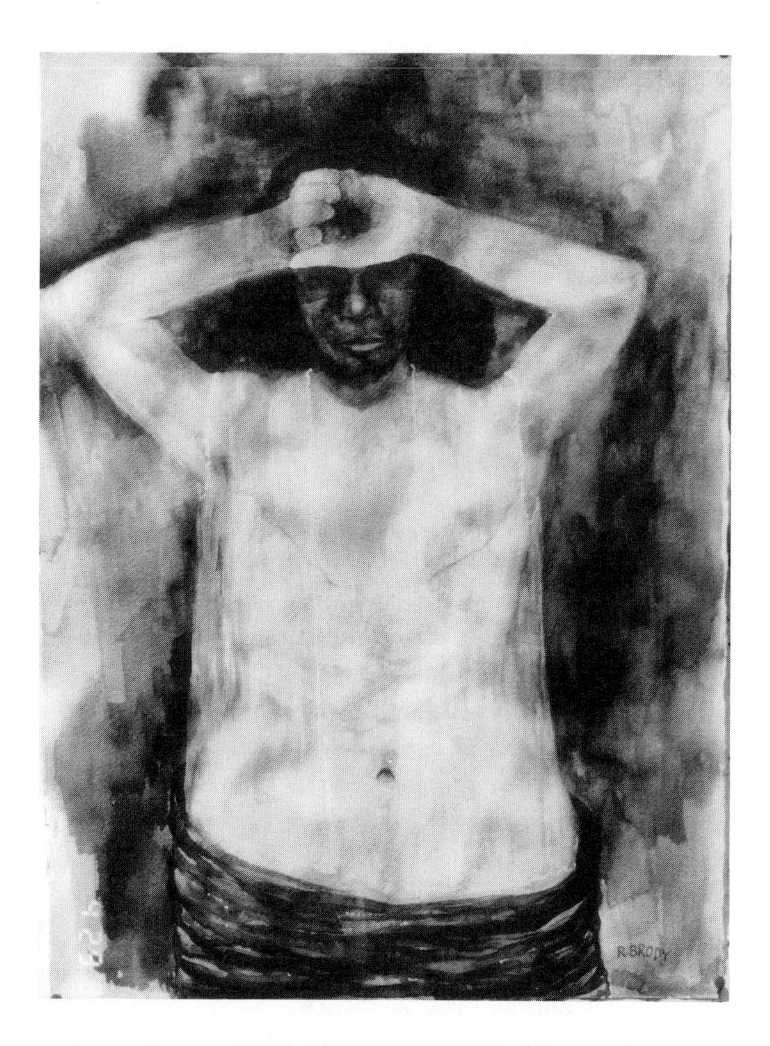

Self Portrait with Double Mastectomy
Ruth Brody, Bronx, New York
Watercolor, 22" x 30", 1993

"My bout with cancer of the breast progressed slowly and methodically—baseline mammogram in my forties, annual mammograms until my sixties when I discovered a lump on self-examination. This turned out to be benign, according to my oncologist. Thereafter, for a number of years, I had semi-annual evaluations eventually leading to needle biopsies, second opinion evaluations and finally the inevitable—double mastectomy at age 73 in June 1990."

Since my insurance company categorized mastectomy as elective surgery, this indicated to me that a difference of opinion exists about the urgency of breast surgery. Elective surgery means that the operation is not a response to a life-or-death situation. Yet doctors and patients often react to a breast-cancer diagnosis as though it becomes worse by the minute, and they buy into the newest treatment finding without realizing that doctors have been rushing their patients into "the newest treatment" for half a century with little improvement in predictable results.

EVALUATING SURGICAL OPTIONS AND TECHNIQUES

One surgical option is *wide excision:* removal of the lump and the surrounding tissue to get clear margins. Although this is sometimes called a *lumpectomy,* technically a lumpectomy does not include any surrounding tissue or lymph nodes; more and more doctors are careful to avoid using the term *lumpectomy* interchangeably with this more extensive conservation surgery.

Dr. Douglas Marchant emphasizes a new element in conservation surgery at the New England Medical Center in Boston. Marchant not only tries to save breasts but strives to give women attractive cosmetic results. He stresses the importance of marking the incision while the patient is still upright. The direction of the incision should follow the natural droop of the breast in the upright position. This simple consideration of the effects of gravity on the incision could make the difference between a salvaged breast and a work of art.[7]

A *partial mastectomy* includes removal of a quadrant of the breast and some lymph nodes. Removal of level-one and -two lymph nodes—the nodes closest to the surface of the armpit—often does not result in arm swelling and, if done with care, should not result in numbness in the underarm tissue.

A *modified radical mastectomy* involves removing all the breast tissue, including the nipple and the skin directly above the tumor, as well as the lymph nodes. It differs from a *radical mastectomy* in that no muscle or chest-wall tissue is removed. A *simple* or *total mastectomy* removes the breast tissue only, no lymph nodes. Some surgeons still encourage mastectomy over lumpectomy. It is up to the patient to find out why a surgeon has made a particular recommendation.

The surgeon is responsible for providing the least mutilating and life-endangering outcome. Many options need to be evaluated and discussed. The device used for incision may be a scalpel, point cauterizer, or laser. The instrument used will affect blood loss and the potential for nerve damage. Lasers, although the most precise of the tools for incision, have some drawbacks. The most serious are that (1) this option is not available at all surgical centers, (2) few doctors are skilled in the technique, and (3) special care must be taken to avoid contact between the laser beam and the anesthesia environment, which is volatile.[8]

One quick way to assess a surgeon's technique is to find out whether he or she regularly uses transfusions for a single mastectomy. When a surgeon's technique is meticulous, a transfusion should not be required. For a bilateral mastectomy, time should be allowed for the patient to put aside her own blood, called autologous blood, for a transfusion. Usually one unit is required.

Surgeons use different techniques to close off the blood vessels: cauterization or tying off. If poorly done, these procedures can result in hematoma, or accumulation of blood under the skin. It is unlikely that a patient can talk a doctor into changing his or her favored approach. If the patient has a preference, then she will need to find a doctor who regularly uses that technique. Once I heard a doctor describe his technique of tying off the blood vessels, I felt that he provided his patients with extraordinary care, although this process is slower than cauterization.

The wound closure is critical to the cosmetic result. Depending on the type of result desired, surgeons can use removable or dissolvable sutures or staples. Removable sutures require a special trip to the surgeon to take them out. Most patients would prefer to avoid this inconvenience and discomfort, but one reason plastic surgeons get such good results is that they do not use dissolvable sutures. Removable sutures hold the wound closed longer than dissolvable sutures do. Adhesive butterfly closures are not a substitute in any area that is likely to be stretched or strained. Most tape is removed a few weeks after surgery to avoid skin irritation.

Approximately six weeks after my surgery, after I started feeling pretty good and began resuming my regular activities, my incision began to spread, causing a wider scar. What had been a fine line became an irregular, keloid-like scar. Everything looked so perfect for the first month that I didn't expect things to change six weeks later. But skin takes a long time to heal, and to achieve an invisible scar, dissolvable sutures may be inadequate.

Staples are obviously the least desirable method for closure, and I would personally avoid any doctor who uses staples on a woman's chest, just on general principle. Staples create an uneven scar and also have to be removed. Ouch!

The dressing—which may be tape or pressure dressing with an Ace bandage—also influences the incidence of hematoma and the patient's general comfort after surgery. Tape can be sticky. Some people are allergic to tape, which can cause itching or a rash. A pressure dressing feels like a bra; the gauze padding provides added protection to the sensitive chest area and is easy to change.

Once the breast tissue has been removed, it is desirable to get as much "grading" information as possible. Several different pathology tests can be ordered. Some hospitals are more likely to run some tests over others. Unfortunately there is no one test that provides the kind of information needed. Does this patient need chemotherapy? What is her chance of having a recurrence? The surgeon and the oncologist should be asked what pathology tests will be performed and what they will learn from these tests.

The oncologist not only should be part of the recovery team but also should see the patient before surgery. There are still surgeons who do not invite oncologists to see their patients before surgery, but I had learned from my mother's cancer experience that the oncologist must be selected as soon as a woman knows she is dealing with cancer. Some protocols recommend chemotherapy before surgery to reduce the size of the tumor, therefore requiring the removal of less tissue. This option cannot be considered if the patient doesn't see the oncologist until after surgery.

ANESTHESIA

If a patient is having general anesthesia, some hospitals will arrange for her to meet with the anesthesiologist before surgery. This doctor is as important as the surgeon. The anesthesiologist is responsible for more than keeping the patient asleep; often he or she also regulates the pain medication, blood transfusions, and other intravenous procedures.

For the convenience of some institutions, anesthesiologists are randomly assigned to operating rooms. It's like catching a cab at the airport—you get the next one in line. A patient who wants to know who this person will be can insist on having the doctor make the selection and set up a meeting prior to the day of surgery.

Local anesthesia has several advantages. The patient can eat before surgery, there isn't any nausea associated with local anesthesia; and only the area to be operated on is anesthetized. Another big advantage is that it can enable the procedure to be done as outpatient surgery. The disadvantage is that the doctor has a limited amount of time to complete work before the anesthesia wears off; in my case, that turned out to be about ten minutes—not adequate time to perform a biopsy, let alone a mastectomy.

I have heard that some facilities are set up so that a patient can have general anesthesia and still be discharged the same day. This should be possible for a biopsy procedure as well. The major drawbacks of general anesthesia are that it is both more risky (it can cause side effects as serious as heart failure) and more costly.

LYMPH NODES

If no lymph nodes are enlarged and causing discomfort, you can choose to not have them removed. I had my lymph nodes removed from only one side, since I was aware that removal is not known to directly affect survival and can result in many physical side effects.

The number and location of removed lymph nodes can have a dramatic effect on mobility and swelling. Depending on the location of the tumor mass and the type of procedure you elect, a second incision—particularly with a lumpectomy—may be required to remove the lymph nodes.

Removal of lymph nodes for diagnostic and staging purposes remains an archaic procedure. If more women complain about this manner of testing, a better technique will be developed. Pathologists need the financial support and incentive to perfect another means of diagnosing spread, such as a tumor marker. For example, prostate cancer can now be determined by a simple blood test, and blood tests are already being performed in Austria and Israel to identify a specific tumor by-product that is associated with early-stage breast cancer.[9] It seems reasonable to suppose that other by-products must be evident in the blood of women who have cancers in more advanced stages.

The formality of removing nodes may give doctors more ammunition to persuade reluctant patients to participate in clinical trials, or it may

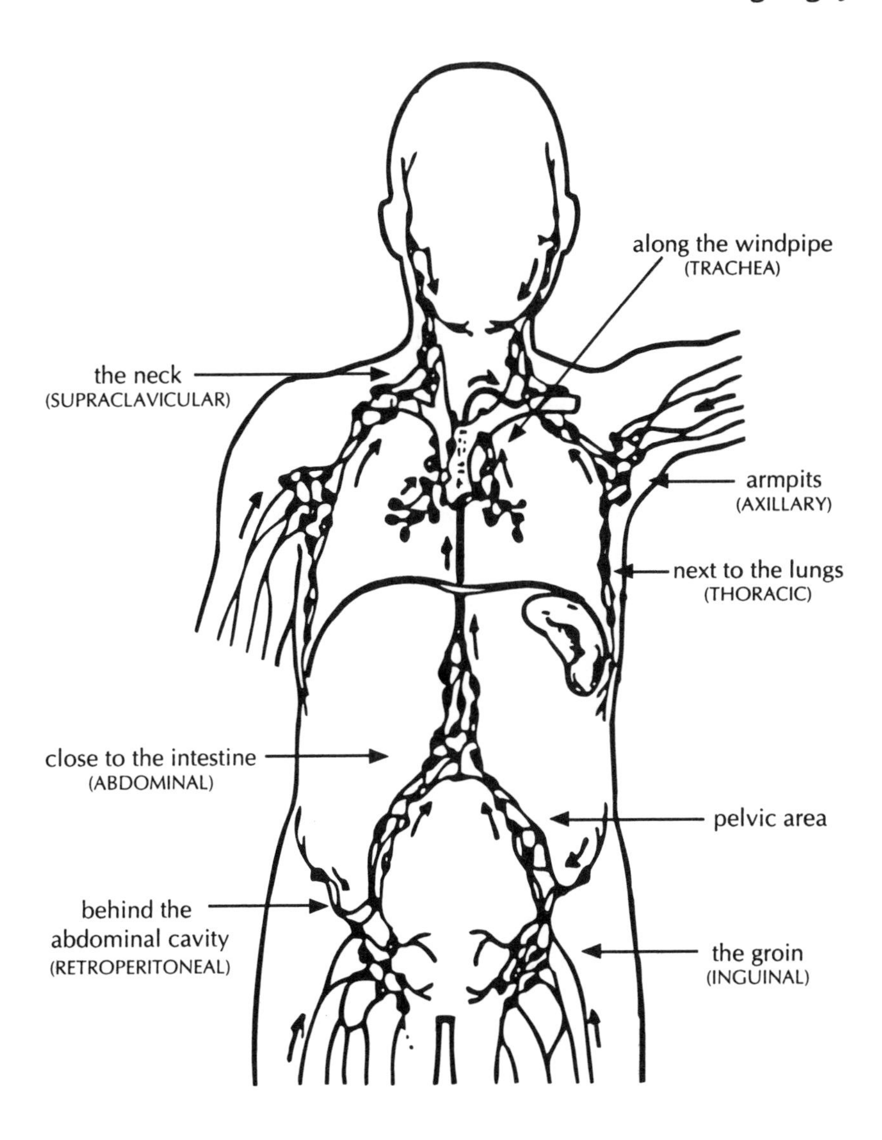

FIGURE 3

THE NORMAL LYMPHATIC SYSTEM

From Saskia R. J. Thiadens, R.N.,
An Information Booklet. National Lymphedema Network.

allow doctors to "stage" each patient according to established standards so that treatment results can be compared with historical results (when lymph nodes were removed without the patient's being given a choice). John Russo, director of the Michigan Cancer Foundation in Detroit and a member of the National Institutes of Health consensus panel on breast-cancer therapy, urges every woman with breast cancer to participate in a clinical trial. "Only ten percent of younger women and only five percent of older women with breast cancer even respond to adjuvant therapy. And there are enough unanswered questions that women would have nothing to lose by entering clinical trials."[10] One breast-cancer survivor asks, "What do they need to remove our lymph nodes for, if they want everyone to be on chemotherapy anyway?"

The removal of lymph nodes is actually one of the more delicate aspects of breast-cancer surgery, and it can result in greater risk as well as discomfort. Lymph-node removal is so delicate because two nerves, the thoracodorsal and the long thoracic nerve (a motor nerve), occupy this same area. Some surgeons don't even try to avoid severing these nerves, aware that some nerve damage is likely to result regardless of how careful they are. This lack of sensitivity by the surgeon results in a permanent lack of sensation in the underarm of the patient.

Muscle damage is also a risk. But the most common complication is swelling—called *edema*—of the arm, underarm, or chest wall. This can result soon after surgery or even years later because of a block in the ability of the lymph system to drain naturally. This problem is often associated with carrying heavy objects, such as a suitcase, or it may develop from an infection that enters through a cut in the affected arm or hand. Exercises and massage (explained in the next chapter,"Treatment Alternatives") may help to relieve these kinds of problems.

Most women do not receive adequate information about the consequences of lymph-node removal. Some doctors are reluctant to discuss the risks, suggesting that if a patient is told about the risks she might become too afraid to consent to the procedure or "confused" by "too much" information. Perhaps someday a research scientist will conduct a study to determine whether ignorance actually has any medical benefit, but I can't imagine that under any circumstance being only half informed could be better than being well-informed. (For information on a patient's rights, see Appendix 4.)

PROSTHESIS OR RECONSTRUCTION

Breast removal creates more than a cosmetic, sexual, self-esteem, or even body-image problem. It is a significant physical alteration without the promise of survival.

Replacing our missing breasts can have more than a cosmetic purpose. Either the prosthesis or the implant provides padding for the rib cage and compensates for the shift in weight distribution to achieve proper body alignment. Breast removal can have a profound effect on our posture. I have been told by women who fit prostheses that a woman with one breast removed runs the risk of developing a pronounced scoliosis if she does not have reconstruction or wear a prosthesis.

Breast surgery is traumatic and an insult to a very sensitive area of the body. After surgery, many women rotate their shoulders in, causing the chest to cave in ever so slightly. This position provides a type of psychological protection, but it does little for the spine or for a woman's overall appearance.

From the first time the doctor mentioned the word *mastectomy,* I decided that having only my left breast removed would be more difficult than losing both. I chose to have my second breast removed because I did not want to have either radiation or chemotherapy. I did not want to expose my weakened immune system to these new carcinogens. And having my second breast removed only required a "simple" mastectomy: no lymph nodes would be removed, making the procedure much easier.

Before my breasts were removed I wondered what I would look like. *Would I hate what I saw?* A good friend offered me her viewpoint a few days before I went to the hospital: "You'll come out looking like a nine-year-old, and it's going to be okay." Fear of the unknown can cause us to imagine results many times worse than the actual result.

Asking plastic surgeons for their professional opinions did not provide me with the type of information I was seeking. One female surgeon said my chest would be caved in, not flat like a child. A male surgeon said I would probably be happier with "bumps" on my chest. I asked both if they had ever put nipples on a flat chest. My desire was to have a finished look rather than a deformed result. If I was going to look like a nine-year-old, perhaps having nipples would make me look less deformed and more whole. The doctors I spoke to had never heard of nor considered such an approach. One surgeon expressed concern that I might come

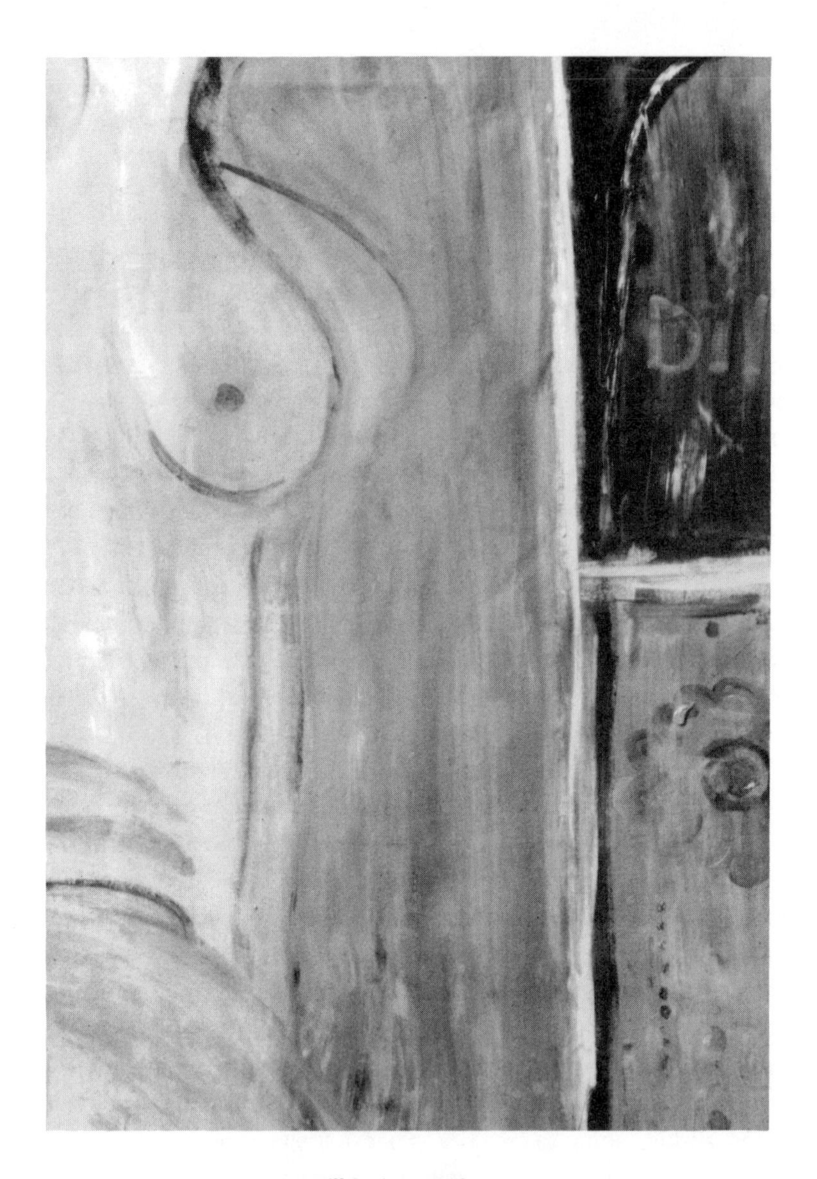

Still Saying Good-Bye
Judith Hoersting, Anchorage, Alaska
Acrylic on canvas, 32" x 24", 1992

"I cried the whole time I painted this. I used a plastic mannequin as my model. I thought, 'I have plastic breasts just like it does.' Finally it came to me: she didn't care, why should I? The dummy taught me something!"

back later and want "bumps," and then the nipples might be in the wrong place.

Not knowing what I would look like made it almost impossible for me to decide whether to have immediate reconstruction. I had always thought that reconstruction was the way to go, especially after seeing the badly deformed chest of a friend who had had a radical mastectomy thirteen years earlier. Her chest was "beyond repair"; since so much tissue had been removed there was no possibility of reconstruction. This image left an imprint on my mind of the worst example of a mastectomy.

While I was weighing reconstruction options, the Food and Drug Administration had already issued a call for the manufacturers to conduct tests on the safety of silicone breast implants. To this day women still have to decide whether to use implants without the benefit of scientific studies that validate their safety. Asking for information where none exists is like asking if there is life on other planets. Because no one really knows, no one can deny the possibility.

I asked about saline implants, but the three surgeons I saw discouraged this option, because of the failure rate and the fact that the saline is placed in a silicone envelope anyway. They told me that silicone implants were safe. Nonetheless, reports were surfacing in the newspaper about women who had become arthritic or stricken with autoimmune disease because of their silicone implants. Even though the final report wasn't in, I felt that I could not put something potentially dangerous into my body as long as I was working so hard to strengthen my health. I did not want to be one of the last women to receive an implant before they were pulled off the market. The other reconstruction options weren't any more promising.

Since April 1991, when I decided not to have reconstruction, two implant manufacturers have withdrawn their silicone products from the market; the FDA called for a moratorium (January 1992) on silicone implants; and a few months later the FDA's advisory panel recommended that the use of silicone implants be limited to "controlled research studies" for women who have mastectomies for cancer. Now, two years later, manufacturers of silicone implants are finalizing a settlement that will create a fund totaling $4.75 billion to compensate women who suffered injuries from having silicone breast implants.

Literally hundreds of articles have been published on this highly emotional subject. Women who feel this form of reconstruction is their only option for wholeness are fighting for access and the right to decide whether they want to take this risk. At the same time, women who have developed body-deforming autoimmune diseases feel that they have been misled about the safety of this product and are suing their doctors and the manufacturers. The Associated Press in February 1992 reported, "Silicone gel breast implants leak much more often than previously believed. . . . Even in implants that don't break open, silicone gel can 'bleed' through the [silicone] casing that encloses the implant."[11]

I question the ethics of leaving the patient responsible for evaluating the safety of a product, and I question the logic of using implants in women who have mastectomies for breast cancer when this is the very population that already has a compromised immune system. These are the women who require regular follow-up mammograms to detect recurrence and who may require other therapies and tests that the implants may interfere with. Unfortunately, data are not yet available that might help us determine whether women who have implants have a higher mortality than women who don't.

I happened to meet with a plastic surgeon who had a glass table in her office. When she handed me a sample of the implant, I put it down on the table for a few minutes and then picked it up again. The implant left a film on the table. Observing this "bleed" effect in just a few minutes' time, I was convinced that silicone was not a stable material and probably didn't stay in the envelope. I was fortunate to have witnessed this effect with my own eyes eight months before the FDA made its decision. The next round of investigations by the FDA will be concerned with saline implants; however, this has not progressed as rapidly as was originally planned. The silicone breast implants were removed on the grounds that their "safety had not been proven," and studies are now being conducted. This left saline the only remaining substitute for women who needed to have their silicone implants removed. Perhaps the industry was able to convince the FDA to slow down their investigation on the saline while the silicone study proceeded. At this time it is unclear how long it will take to adequately study the use of silicone in the human body. The fact that they were used for 30 years without investigation could be an indication that both economic and political factors have more influence on safety than anyone would like to believe.

ALTERNATIVES TO SYNTHETIC IMPLANTS

One plastic surgeon spent a great deal of time giving me the sales pitch on having double *abdominal flap* reconstruction. After completing his sales pitch, he examined my abdomen and discovered that I did not have enough fatty tissue for this procedure. It was no wonder, since I had been doing sit-ups regularly for the past six months. And I had serious reservations about this procedure, since I still wanted the option of having a baby some day. I was concerned that if my abdominal muscles were to be moved up to my chest, I might not be able to support a womb. When the surgeon insisted that even carrying a baby would be possible, I knew I was getting a hard sell.

Other implant techniques that are available include the *latissimus dorsi flap,* which utilizes one of the back muscles that is normally used for shoulder movement. This procedure does not result in a very large mound, and a synthetic implant is often required. The most complex reconstructive surgery is the free flap. What initially sounds like a perfect solution—taking muscle, skin, and fat from the buttocks and placing it on the chest wall—is highly complex because the blood supply must also be reconnected, requiring delicate vascular surgery.

All these methods require more than one surgical procedure to restore the breast mound. All create additional scars on the body. Even when synthetic implants are inserted at the time of the mastectomy, this is not a one-step procedure. Several different approaches are used. The plastic surgeons all agreed on one thing—a reconstructed breast never looks the same as a natural breast. I heard this loud and clear. Even a bump or a mound—or whatever they choose to call it—isn't and will never be just like my breast.

It is difficult to position a reconstructed breast and get it to droop. One surgeon told me he had mastered a technique for accomplishing a droop. Following the mastectomy operation an inflatable implant is inserted under the chest muscle. This temporary implant, called a tissue expander, is then expanded gradually over a few months. A small port allows the surgeon to add saline solution to the implant.

Once the mound reaches the desired size, the size is noted; however, the doctor continues to add more and more saline until the mound is two to three times larger than the woman actually wants it to be. This is done to stretch the skin. I was told that the doctor who invented this process observed the skin-expanding ability of a pregnant woman's belly and translated his observation into breast expansion.

Once the expander reaches this exaggerated limit, the patient continues to wear it around for another few months. Then, in a second surgical procedure, the tissue expander is removed and the chosen-size "permanent" implant is inserted. Since the skin was stretched beyond what is required, the final result is a droop. The nipple is constructed during a third operation—possibly with only a local anesthetic—and the areola is tattooed to produce a darkened area.

This sounded like an excellent solution, but I found out that as with all types of implant surgery, problems can arise. The body can be allergic to some or all of the substances used. The tissue can become cut off from the blood supply and die. It is natural for the body to try to reject the implant, which causes an infection and requires antibiotics. Scar tissue typically forms around the implant in an attempt to seal off this foreign substance. This scar tissue can become tight and constrict the implant, causing discomfort. Implants can develop leaks or become broken under certain circumstances. Even in implants that do not leak, sweating or seeping occurs through the envelope, as I have already described.

Women, breast-cancer organizations, politicians, and plastic surgeons fought to keep silicone implants on the market for economic and emotional reasons. They said that taking implants off the market takes away women's "right to choose." What kind of choice is it for women to feel so compelled to endanger their health? This public debate helped to demonstrate the social conditioning women receive. Many women came to the FDA hearing to say that the implants changed their lives for the better. More implant users are women who opt for this procedure strictly for augmentation.

To make my final decision about reconstruction, in addition to visiting plastic surgeons, I visited stores that sold prostheses and was surprised to learn that I was the first person to have ever come in *before* surgery. I wondered how anyone could make an informed decision without looking at the prosthesis.

The appearance of the prosthesis is clearly not a selling factor. Perhaps because many young women opt for reconstruction, the prosthesis market is primarily targeted toward older, large-breasted women. Perhaps the manufacturers have just lost touch with their clientele. But by visiting the local medical-supply store, I discovered that the prostheses available to women who have mastectomies is pretty dismal. The prosthesis, despite being an alternative to more surgery, scars, and medical bills, is almost as unacceptable as the potentially harmful silicone implant.

Thinking through all my options and possible outcomes in the days before my surgery helped me stay calm for a while. The night before was the most difficult. My foremost fear was that afterwards I wouldn't recover, and my health would just slip away. But I had carefully chosen my surgeon. When the morning of surgery arrived and I felt reduced to a terrified little child, not knowing what I would look like twenty-four hours later, my doctor was both gentle and sympathetic.

Bredenberg recommends that "a simple drawing of the scar" provides women with "anticipatory imaging" prior to the operation. Looking at medical books that described the surgery helped me to envision my new figure. After the surgery, my doctor let me decide when I was ready to see the result. I chose to see myself for the first time in a private examination room with a door, away from family members and nursing intrusions.

Initially, I had decided on a prosthesis, and I wanted one that felt like me, one that was not heavy and did not add weight to my shoulders. I wanted a prosthesis that was soft and felt good against my skin, not hot and gel-like. I needed a secure prosthesis that would not move around in an aerobics class or swimming pool. I did not want to be embarassed by a floating boob! I wanted to be able to wear all the same clothes I did before—silk blouses and pullover sweaters make me feel sexy, so I searched for a prosthesis that fit my particular needs. Eventually, I decided to make my own, which I now understand is *not* uncommon. This is another area in need of change, where women need to speak up about their dissatisfaction. After the initial adjustment I soon switched to cotton T-shirts and abandoned my homemade prosthesis.

Now that I can look back on my choice, I'm very satisfied with the results. My chest isn't caved in; it has two scars, but it is flat, just like that of a nine-year-old. I like having the option of going braless, and most of the time I do. Some people who don't know I had surgery have remarked, "You look great. Have you lost weight?"

REHABILITATION

In the future, I would like to see a comprehensive rehabilitation program for women with breast cancer. I needed to rehabilitate myself emotion-

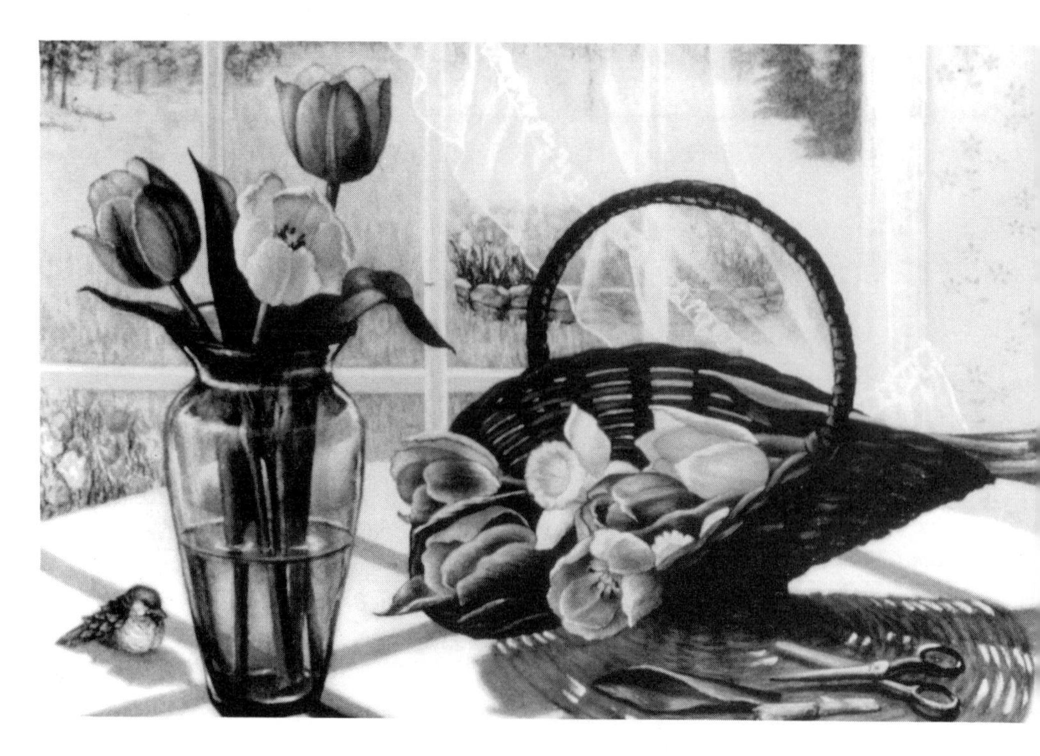

From My Garden
Camille Cote Beaupre, Monroe, Connecticut
Pastel, 24" x 30", 1992

"I have always taken great pleasure in living and have been a very active, healthy person. Though cancer had taken the lives of both my parents as well as that of their brothers and sister, I chose not to dwell on the thought. However, I did take the precautions of having a complete yearly physical as well as exercising daily and living as healthfully as I possibly could. I was completely taken aback, therefore, by the diagnosis of breast cancer at 59, and by the radical mastectomy and year of chemotherapy that followed. It was then that I realized what a tremendous gift life is, and also how fragile it is."

---

ally, physically, and spiritually, and I had to do this by going to a variety of practitioners and paying for these services out of my own resources.

The only community-based outreach programs are staffed by volunteers. Limited information is available for women about adjusting to this new body image and to the emotional issues that surround breast cancer. The American Cancer Society's "Reach for Recovery" program has attempted to address physical rehabilitation, but the volunteers, however well-meaning, sometimes impart inaccurate information.

Rehabilitation education means education about diet, physical exercise, and movement as well as opportunities for a woman to become self-confident with her new shape and to talk openly about her concerns. Rehabilitation should include massage, acupuncture, and yoga. Rehabilitation is whatever it takes to restore health to what it was before surgery—or even better.

Rehabilitation programs need to be consistent with a patient's needs. Women who have bilateral mastectomies require a different program from those who have had less extensive breast surgery. Having lymph nodes removed on both sides causes many new challenges during the first six months. Oncology nurses have an opportunity to assist the recovery process, but they too need to be trained in handling the whole range of breast-cancer patients' special needs with an open mind. Patients need encouragement to fight for their lives. Instead, they are often told to just resume their former activities and act as though nothing had happened. Medical personnel discourage macrobiotic diets as "radical" and dangerous without offering any alternative suggestions.

Exercise programs need to become an integral part of breast-cancer treatment. Women deserve a formalized recovery program. To get it, we need the funds to study the advantages of specific rehabilitation programs. The National Cancer Institute reports that a paltry 1 percent of the breast-cancer research budget is given to rehabilitation research. This area has been grossly neglected. Doctors need justification to recommend that these programs be incorporated in cancer clinics and health centers. Insurance companies will not provide reimbursement without doctor referrals and controls.

Recovery from breast cancer presents some unique problems. Yet, this need remains underserved. Because a woman's arm mobility may be impaired as a result of the surgery, activities she used to take for granted—like tennis or golf, or even lifting her own suitcase—may no longer be possible. A woman's posture can be affected even if she has only had a lumpectomy. A rehabilitation program for women with breast cancer should be graduated for women with special needs and limitations. The sooner rehabilitation is started after surgery, the less likely a woman will be to develop poor posture and atrophied muscle extension.

At first, stretching, pool exercises, and manual lymph drainage (a type of massage that focuses on the lymphatic system) both support and soften the mending tissues. The natural tendency is to favor a traumatized area, but this only compounds the problem of contracted muscles and scar tissue. Shoulder and breathing exercises that open up and expand the chest cavity—on a regular, do-what-you-can basis—benefit posture, mobility, and self-esteem. I dream about the day when every woman who undergoes breast surgery receives rehabilitation therapy as a normal protocol.

The strength in my left arm—the side from which I had lymph nodes removed—decreased after surgery. I am prone to slight lymphedema and have diminished ability to perspire on that side. Because of the careful surgical technique, however, I regained almost all of my underarm sensation and contour. Many women aren't so fortunate with mobility and appearance.

My ability to lift suitcases, push down casement windows, or engage in some types of weight-bearing exercise has been affected. Doctors vary in their recommendations about how long a patient should wait before carrying heavy objects after lymph-node removal. My surgeon told me that I had no restrictions and should start swimming daily three weeks after surgery. Several women I know who have regained all mobility used swimming to help themselves rehabilitate. I was taking golf lessons three months after surgery; I think my golf swing has actually improved!

I spent time looking at myself in the mirror and really getting comfortable with my new chest. Sometimes I completely forget I had surgery; my chest feels completely whole and normal. My surgeon took the time and care to provide me with a special result.

My desire was to become so completely comfortable with my body that I could strip nude at the health club or even sunbathe topless. I was always jealous of men not having to wear bras, and it sometimes seemed odd to me that women have to cover their chests when men don't.

Apparently I am not the only woman who has pondered this distinction. In 1991, ten to fifteen women bared their breasts and marched through the town of Brattleboro, Vermont, calling for freedom of expression for women. They protested because women's breasts are considered obscene—men can go topless without punishment, but women cannot.

The double standard is that breasts are nonetheless exploited—displayed and discussed in most public situations. No one restricts reconstructed breasts from appearing in full color in *Time* magazine. In order for a movie to be successful it is believed that it must have "T and A"—tits and ass. Yet until Anita Hill confronted Clarence Thomas on national television, using the word *penis* on TV was considered taboo. Opposition raged over TV advertising about the use of condoms for safe sex, but no one restricts the advertisement of bras and mammograms. *Lear's* magazine says that breasts more than any other part of our bodies, have been glorified, "eroticized, analyzed, and even politicized." Breasts are exposed as art, symbolized in poetry, dramatized in theater. Both men and women accept the exploitation of the breast. And both sexes become equally uncomfortable when the same attention is directed toward the penis.

Breasts seem to get everyone's interest—that is, until they are cut into and off by the thousands. Few people feel comfortable thinking about that. Women get many mixed messages: some husbands refuse to look at their wives after surgery, some doctors cause women to feel they are narcissistic to want reconstruction after amputation, other doctors don't feel they have done a good job if a woman doesn't have reconstruction, and everyone tries to encourage women who have had mastectomies to wear a prosthesis. If society is so hung up on breasts, why aren't people demanding better surgical options for women with breast cancer? Why are so many mastectomies still being performed?[12] Are there other women out there who would rather have amputation than toxic cocktails and radiation? Is the treatment for breast cancer just another form of exploitation of women?

No one is able to explain why mastectomies or more invasive operations continue to be performed despite clear proof that they do not influence disease-free survival.[13] Perhaps women themselves are less hung up about their breasts than they are about survival. I've heard many women say, "If they told me that having my breast removed would mean

I no longer had cancer, I would say fine, I'll do that. But the truth is they say, 'We have to remove your breast and we can't guarantee you that this will save your life.'" That's what makes this sacrifice so difficult. There is no guaranteed outcome, even if you consent to the treatment. For me, having a mastectomy meant I made the choice to give up my breasts because doing so would buy me some more time to find wholeness and health.

Ultimately, whether or not they are facing breast surgery, women need to be able to say: "I'm okay—with breasts, without breasts, with a bra, without a bra. I'm not my breasts, and my body and breasts aren't objects."

7

Treatment Alternatives

A healing technique is a vehicle for connecting with another person in a certain way that promotes the movement toward wholeness. Each of us has a technique—perhaps several—that has to do, in some way, with our personality.

Rachel Naomi Remen, M.D., F.A.A.P.

Through the entire healing process I attempted to balance the idea of treatment with the process of boosting my immune system and reversing the damage that had caused the cancer to develop in the first place. I started immediately after diagnosis by changing my diet. From this point on, many other possibilities opened up: herbs, supplements, energy balancing, bodywork. Once people heard about how I was trying to heal my cancer, they would tell me stories about other people who had seemingly miraculous cures or who had lost their lives in spite of their courage to try other treatments. I also heard of people who died praying for God to take away the cancer, while others told me how God spared someone they knew.

On some level I knew if I tried to "do everything" I would run the risk of exhausting my immune system and possibly my spirit. Therefore, I had to choose from the vast array of alternative treatments available. I looked for treatments that reflected my view of cancer, which is that cancer is a symptom of a larger problem. The tumor and all the cellular changes that go along with it are symptoms of a poorly functioning immune system. Every treatment offered by traditional medicine is designed to remove, suppress, counteract, deplete, or replace the conditions that result from and are labeled as cancer. My response was to treat my whole body and not just the symptoms.

Seeing a practitioner who was skilled in Oriental diagnosis—through taking my pulse and looking at my face, tongue, hands, and ears—provided me with an alternative method of determining how strong my overall system was. Early on I adopted the approach of using three methods of assessment: traditional diagnostic procedures (bone scans, chest x-rays, mammograms, and blood tests), Oriental evaluations, and intuitive assessments. I wanted to develop and learn to trust my own barometer of how I was, rather than rely solely on what other people saw with their methods of evaluating health and disease.

Finding ways to harmonize the different energies in and around my body meant trying a variety of techniques and adjusting my program according to my condition. I sought to

1. Strengthen and purify my blood with herbs and vitamins.
2. Improve my circulation and strengthen my tissues and organs with exercise, massage, and herbs. At first I was only able to do gentle exercises like yoga; later I adopted aerobics, weight training, and Quigong.
3. Open up blocked energy meridians with acupuncture treatments, Reiki, and shiatsu.
4. Improve my digestion and food absorption with diet, herbs, and vitamins.

All these complementary therapies worked to restore my whole system and prepare my body for the long term. When surgery eventually became necessary, I had already been on an immune-system-building program for two years. Much of the old fat and toxins had already been removed. My liver, spleen, and kidneys, although under stress from coping with the cancer, were functioning in the best manner possible. I felt that I went into surgery far healthier than at the time of diagnosis; I also gained many new tools and learned how to listen to my body. When it was determined after surgery that I had five positive lymph nodes, I decided to consider alternative drug therapies. Even though at this juncture I needed to add something much stronger to my treatment, I still

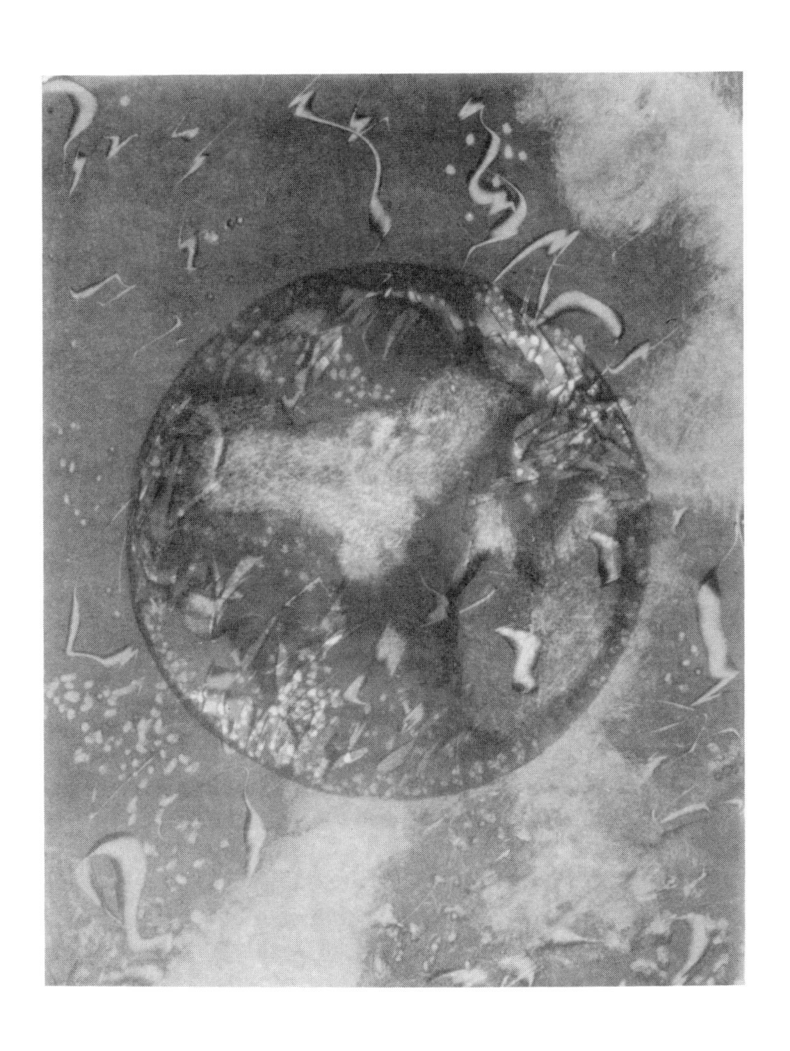

The Beginning
Mary Knoll Ahacic, Arlington, Ohio
Monotype, 29" x 23", 1990

"My artwork served as a catalyst to sort out this life-threatening disease, its consequences, and my new response to the world. . . . It helped me to understand the disease on my terms rather than on its terms. Because I didn't know whether I'd be alive after one year, my artwork became a high priority. Also, I hoped it would serve as a memoir."

made choices that fit my criteria of therapies that would attack the cancer without compromising my immune system. At this stage I didn't want to poison my cells and my system.

It wasn't until after surgery that I decided to investigate chemical systemic treatments. My approach was to start with the gentlest forms and reconsider incorporating more aggressive treatments if they became necessary. Only when the benefits were appropriate to my circumstance and the risks not detrimental to my immune system would I add a new treatment. Everything needed to have a time and a purpose.

Unlike the traditional medical approach to cancer treatment, my adjuvant therapies had to do more than attack the cancer; they had to enhance the health of my body and spirit. I found herbs, acupuncture, home remedies, yoga, Quigong, manual lymph drainage, vitamins, and 714X to be truly holistic because they all possessed strengthening and energy-balancing properties.

HERBS

My herb formulas were provided by a person trained in the use of Oriental herbs. These special formulas were made up for my particular condition every week. I also received instructions about how to prepare them: for instance, herbs in pure water, not tap, are simmered for an hour or so to make a heavy black tea. These medicinal herb drinks helped me to increase my energy, eliminate better, and menstruate without PMS. They even resulted in my blood samples changing color—from dark red to purple to bright red.

Bark, seeds, roots, mushrooms, and berries were all combined to make up my special formula. If my bowel movements became too soft or too hard the formula was changed accordingly.

I drank my herbs every day—twice a day during the first six months after my diagnosis. After that I drank them periodically to correct or strengthen a particular condition, such as a weak spleen, toxic kidneys, or congested lungs; to prepare my body for surgery; and to aid my recovery from surgery. The herbs helped me regain my strength by removing the toxins from my system or adding what my system needed. If a blood test, for example, indicated I was low in iron, then the herbs were adjusted until this condition disappeared, which surprisingly might take just a few days. Initially these thick dark brown teas reminded me more of sludge than of anything I might want to drink, but once I became accustomed to the potent formulas, I actually enjoyed drinking them because they gave me an energy boost. If I happened to miss one serving I would notice the fatigue.

ACUPUNCTURE

The health counselor who provided the herbs also offered acupuncture treatments. I found out I was very responsive to acupuncture. Most of the treatments involved placing needles in my ankles; some treatments were also in my wrists. A second acupuncturist I saw preferred doing treatments in his patients' hands with extremely fine nondisposable needles.

The hand treatments were difficult for me. Having approximately fifteen needles inserted in my palms, on my fingers, and on the backs of my hands was both psychologically and physically stressful. The needles were inserted while I was lying down, but after the practitioner was finished, I was expected to sit in the lobby area. The needles remained in place for twenty minutes, then each patient removed his or her own needles.

I had several problems with this process. First, these needles were sterilized and reused. Since the AIDS epidemic is a looming concern, and since the practitioner treated people with chronic fatigue syndrome, I wondered about using reusable needles, even if they were sterilized. And because people walked around with these needles in their hands, sometimes a needle would fall onto the floor without anyone's realizing it. Everyone was also expected to remove their shoes upon entering the treatment area, so it was possible that a nonsterilized needle might get stepped on. These conditions made this particular acupuncture center a less-than-desirable treatment facility.

More typically, the person receiving acupuncture remains in a reclining position so that he or she can relax or meditate during the treatment. I found this process more worthwhile. I usually felt invigorated, refreshed, and introspective after a relaxing acupuncture session. Additionally, if I had any aches or pains, a headache, or lower back pain, these problems would vanish during the treatment. This non-drug-oriented therapy convinced me that there is more to pain and symptoms than is commonly understood in the American culture.

HOME REMEDIES

My macrobiotic counselor and acupuncturist exposed me to nondrug treatments known as home remedies. Herbal salves, medications, and teas could be recommended for most conditions—everything from a mosquito bite to a chest cold and after-surgery pain. Simple herbal preparations restored my health without the side effects of antibiotics or pain killers. To this day, if I have any kind of ache, I call my acupuncturist before I call the doctor.

EXERCISE

Regular exercise—anything from yoga to walking, bicycling, swimming, or aerobics—is very complementary to a health-restoring program. What I could do at the time depended on my current physical condition. When I was most ill, just before surgery, my health counselor did not want me to discharge my physical energy. Instead, he instructed me in how to absorb more healing energy with gentle exercises.

His concern was that vigorous exercising like bicycling, swimming, and aerobics would diminish my energy and create chaos. For a while I agreed to direct my healing energy inward. However, as I became healthier I wanted a more vigorous exercise program.

The amount and type of exercise used needs to be tailored to the person's state of health. For instance, many women benefit enormously from swimming after surgery; however, someone who is not used to cardiovascular exercise might find swimming too exhausting. The key is to listen to your own body and do only the amount of exercise that feels appropriate. If you feel tired after exercising, your workout has been too intense; exercise should energize you rather than cause fatigue.

During the time when I suspected that the cancer had spread to my lymph nodes, I tried to work out to burn off excess body fat and burn off the cancer. This approach did not help. Whether the amount of spread was connected to this kind of intense exercising, I can't be certain. But I did notice a change—a change for the worse! Since exercise and heat from a Jacuzzi or sauna stimulate the flow of blood, it seems plausible that they could stimulate tumor growth, which is dependent upon increased blood supply.

YOGA AND QUIGONG

I integrated yoga into my healing program early on. Later, for a more advanced workout, I learned a Chinese martial-art form called Quigong. Both helped me improve my strength and flexibility without draining away my energy. I found these forms of exercise extremely energizing and centering.

I was able to relearn the yoga postures on my own by using Richard Hittleman's *Yoga: 28-Day Exercise Plan.*[1] I got up each morning, put on my yoga clothes, and went into the spare room to practice. Beginning with the exercise recommended for day one, I practiced initially only twenty minutes. In a very short time I was able to practice for forty-five minutes without even realizing how much time had passed.

Quigong was harder to master. I took private instruction and the teacher tailored the exercises to my particular condition. Arm and breathing exercises helped me to keep a clear mind and restore my mobility. I was even able to use this form of exercise the day after my mastectomy as a way to rehabilitate my muscle strength and reach.

LYMPH REHABILITATION

Three weeks after surgery my doctor encouraged me to start swimming. I reluctantly reported to the pool three or four times a week. (A near-drowning incident when I was a child still makes me feel hesitant in the water.) In the beginning I could only flap my arms, or kick my legs while floating on my back. When I tried to take a breast stroke, I felt as though my abdominal muscles had been reconnected to my ribs. For some reason my abdominals were tender for a long while after the surgery. Swimming did, however, significantly increase my mobility.

To improve local lymph function and reduce edema, I found a practitioner experienced in "manual lymph drainage." Once I began manual lymph-drainage treatments—a specialized form of lymph "massage" developed in Europe—I was also able to increase my mobility and swimming therapy. Although it is difficult to describe this technique, lymph-drainage therapy is a very gentle but effective method of simultaneously treating the muscular, nervous, vascular, immune, and lymphatic systems.[2] Lymph drainage is said to stimulate the metabolism, quicken the healing process, reduce and eliminate pain, detoxify the body, and reduce stress. I can truly say I found this claim to be accurate. The

National Lymphedema Network in San Francisco is a professional organization for practitioners skilled in this technique. One way to find a lymph-drainage masseur is through this network, whose address is given in the resources section at the end of this book.

The purpose of this specialized kind of massage after surgery is to soften the scar tissue so that it does not pull the skin taut, to prevent edema, and to improve the circulation around the area of the operation. I was delighted to find that I still had excellent nerve sensation in this area, and I believe that this type of massage greatly facilitated my healing and mobility.

VITAMINS AND DOWSING

To compliment my diet and exercise programs, which I modified as my condition changed, I also took vitamins. The one vitamin that I have taken consistently is vitamin C. Since my diet does not include citrus fruits, I felt I needed to supplement my vitamin C intake. (Citrus grows in warmer climates and is considered by macrobiotic practitioners to have a chilling effect on the body during the winter or at higher latitudes.)

Linus Pauling's famous research demonstrated that vitamin C improves the immune-system function and the mobility of white blood cells. Vitamin C was used in large doses by Norman Cousins[3] when he was fighting his joint inflammation. It is also an antioxidant and scavenger of free radicals.[4] Free radicals are molecules with an odd number of electrons, which seem to promote disease in our bodies. Even though medical schools have courses devoted to pharmacology, vitamin therapy is not included. Because of this void in most doctors' training, they often are unable to advise their patients about the benefits of vitamins and sometimes go so far as to say that supplements have no value. As time has passed the value of vitamins has become more widely acknowledged.

The vitamins and minerals that seem to have a beneficial influence in fighting breast cancer are beta carotene, B-1, B-2, B-6, B-12, D, E, and selenium. Korean ginseng, shark-oil capsules, and enzymes such as bromelain are also recommended for building the immune system.

Instead of taking everything, or too much of one thing and too little of another, I have found that a dowsing pendulum takes the guesswork out of what dose is appropriate in my vitamin therapy. My understanding is that all people have the ability to dowse, but some are more responsive than others. The people I know who dowse seem to have a good sense of humor and an open mind. Vermont happens to be home to the headquarters of the American Society of Dowsers, so it hardly surprises anyone here to see someone dowsing or to hear someone tell a dowsing story.

After surgery and drug therapy, I started my maintenance program: blue-green algae, vitamin C, concentrated liquid beta carotene, and bancha tea (a type of green tea that is very low in caffeine) as daily supplements. Although I had been drinking bancha tea since starting my new way of eating and preparing food, more than two years later the following headline appeared in my local newspaper: "Green Tea Could Help Prevent Cancer, Research Shows." A study at the American Health Foundation found that mice developed "45 percent fewer lung tumors if they drank a 2 percent tea solution instead of water. Researchers think such chemicals inhibit cancer development by scavenging the damaging fragments created when carcinogens break molecules in the body."[5] From this description, it sounds as though green tea also helps to remove free radicals.[6]

A newly released study has put together many of the puzzle pieces about breast cancer—mutagenic changes in DNA, the value of antioxidants, alcohol consumption, environmental contaminants, and increased estrogen. Reseachers from the Pacific Northwest Research Foundation report that their findings provide "important insight into how breast cancer develops." Drs. Donald Malins, Eric Holmes, and Sandra Gunselman, together with Dr. Nayak Polissar, biostatistician at the University of Washington, discovered that "changes in oxygen metabolism in the female breast result in severe damage to the components of DNA (the nucleotide bases) that hold the genetic code. . . . Alterations in the breasts' oxygen metabolism increase free radical concentrations which attack the DNA, producing mutagenic changes that increase the risk of developing cancer." This stress in tissues is known to be reduced by antioxidants, which include vitamin C, vitamin E, and beta carotene. Good sources of these vitamins are broccoli, carrots, and other dark green and orange vegetables and fruits.

The blue-green algae preparation has helped me to digest my food more effectively and to purify my system. Algae is a whole-food supplement, not really a vitamin at all. My diet remains primarily organic, but I am not as fanatic about it as I was for the first year after my diagnosis. If I get a dull headache when I eat something that may have been treated with preservatives or pesticides, I recognize it as my warning signal that the food I'm eating is not clean.

A DRUG: 714X

Six weeks after surgery, I was not regaining my strength. I was worried that the surgery had severely depleted my immune system, and I wanted to find a cell-oriented systemic treatment to help restore my energy and treat the cancer cells that nestled in my lymph system. Diet, herbs, exercise, acupuncture, and vitamins clearly weren't enough; still, I was not convinced that chemotherapy was my best option. The dose is standardized and could not be adjusted to take into account my extreme drug sensitivity.

I discovered the experimental drug 714X in the same way I discovered many other unconventional treatments. People told me about it, and I listened skeptically at first. After several people who had no relationship to each other all mentioned the same treatment, I decided to spend some time researching what 714X could do and how it worked to achieve long-term removal of the cancer cells that remain in the bloodstream.

This drug is injected intralymphatically near the groin with an extremely small tuberculin needle for three twenty-one-day cycles. People who had taken 714X claimed phenomenal success. My only problem was that I needed to either find someone to do the injections for me or learn how to do self-injections, since this is not a drug Americans can obtain at the local hospital or a clinic.

The drug 714X is not illegal, but it is not FDA-approved, either. Doctors can prescribe it and administer it, but most don't want to be responsible for the administration. I was able to find someone who was qualified and agreeable to the time commitment to administer 714X for me; later, I learned to do the injections myself. An out-of-state doctor marked the location for the injections and guided me on how to do them. After three days I started to notice an improvement in my energy and to feel better in many other ways. My color improved, the circulation in my hands and feet improved, and the gloomy, depressed feelings I was having disappeared.

Initially I learned about 714X by reading *The Trial and Persecution of Gaston Naessens* by Christopher Bird. Naessens, a French microbiologist living in Canada, invented a unique microscope that allowed him to develop his own cell theory, and he then created 714X. Naessens believes that there is an "indestructible organism, [called] a somatid or tiny body, that inhabits the fluids of all living things, especially human blood plasma."[8] When the body becomes ill, the blood cycle changes. This is visible in Naessens' microscope but not in a regular dark-field microscope. According to Naessens, this parasitized condition is what contributes to the continuing breakdown of the blood and immune function.

I was able to view my own blood in this special microscope at a doctor's office in the United States. Before the treatment, a sample was taken. I could see that my red blood cells were weak—the outer edges had breaks, and some cells were misshapen and deformed. I could see with my own eyes why I was sick. This was both frightening and exciting.

After completing the three cycles of treatment, I had a follow-up blood test. This time my red blood cells looked strong and well-formed. Only a few cells were misshapen, and I was advised that they would continue to be removed as time progressed, even after I had stopped using the drug.

The microscope test also revealed somatid activity, the activity of the white blood cells, the condition of my liver, and whether I had anemia. A person skilled at interpreting the smear—created by placing a spot of fresh blood on a clean slide—could tell a patient within minutes if his or her health was in peril. Naessens claims that he can diagnose the potential for cancer two years before a tumor is detectable by standard techniques.

The experience made me feel fortunate to have discovered this drug and evaluation technique. Until I had an unanticipated recurrence, my post-operative annual follow-up now consisted of the regular tests that I describe earlier and the Naessens microscope blood test. Unfortunately the microscope did not provide the advance warning I had hoped for, and 714X did not prevent a recurrence.

Some think Naessens is the Galileo of the twentieth century; yet to accept Naessens' theory, mainstream scientists would have to rethink the idea that all microbial life comes from "outside" the body. Naessens postulates that bacteria and yeast-like forms may be created by our own bodies when a deficient internal environment exists. This concept of a parasitic condition fit with other theories I had heard from holistic practitioners. One reason why advanced cancers may be so difficult to treat is a secondary condition that fosters an environment conducive to parasite growth. Drug treatments like chemotherapy can kill cells, but they also create an environment conducive to new parasites, which seem to become more and more unresponsive and immune to the toxic chemicals—much as insects become immune to insecticides.

In 1989 Naessens was tried in Quebec because a woman with advanced breast cancer died after using 714X. The charge was not that the drug actually caused her death but that she didn't take the standard treatment. Naessens was responsible for injecting the drug and was therefore accused of practicing medicine. Naessens survived the legal system and was acquitted by a jury. Anecdotal stories for both the defense and the plaintiff are recounted in Bird's book. For more than fifteen years, Naessens has had a success rate of better than 50 percent in reversing advanced cancers. His success rate is far better than what has been achieved with chemotherapy, and it has none of the undesirable side effects.

The premise on which 714X works is that it provides nitrogen to the cancer cells so they do not feed off the healthy cells and create a toxic environment. Without this toxic discharge, the immune system is able to identify the cancer cells and naturally destroy and discharge them. The internal environment is ultimately restored to a nontoxic condition.

For me, 714X was the ideal drug. It helped me to heal naturally while making me feel better emotionally and look better physically, rather than making me look worse or feel depressed as do so many cancer treatments. (I did not subscribe to the premise that I had to "suffer" to get well.)

Eating a healthy diet and facilitating the purification of the kidneys and colon during this process are also very important. In fact, an informational video provided by Naessens says that diet is 40 percent of the battle. Continuing to eat toxic foods or foods that move through the system slowly would inhibit this drug process.

ALTERNATIVE PRACTITIONERS

One word of caution about treatment alternatives seems both appropriate and necessary. Some people choose to use alternative therapies in conjunction with standard treatment. Others insist that the patient be a purist, using alternative treatment instead of the standard treatment. Every woman must ultimately decide what is appropriate to her own condition and emotional makeup. Using alternative treatments can be slow and disappointing or it can be a miraculous process. Why a given treatment works for one person and not for another remains a mystery. Perhaps the answers are locked in our psyches, where we hold thoughts about our past and future. Whatever we decide is what is right for us. Still, we need the support of others. This is a time when we are most vulnerable to unethical practitioners.

As I explored the vast world of alternative practitioners, I found varying degrees of competence in both licensed and nonlicensed doctors. I met two M.D.s who provided innovative treatments but were also providing second-rate medical care. They were abusing the system in two ways: both as doctors and as alternative practitioners. They tried to see the most people in the shortest amount of time while charging extraordinary fees: two hundred dollars for a twenty-minute consultation. I felt cheated as well as abused.

Additionally, some alternative practitioners aren't 100 percent genuine. They too can abuse the gifts of healing that have been bestowed on them. Taking responsibility for treating cancer patients carries with it the responsibility of recognizing the limitations of the treatments.

In order to "control" his patients and keep them coming back, one healer used his skills with herbs and acupuncture the way a pimp uses drugs. By making his victims "feel good" he convinced his clients that they needed him to survive. Meanwhile, the sick person didn't really improve but had an illusion of well-being. To me, this seemed as criminal as selling illegal drugs. I trusted this person to provide me with the right formula; I did not expect the formula to contain mind-altering substances.

Many of this man's clients came for a three-week residential program. This included room, two meals per day, lessons in yoga and theory, and treatment. Vitamin supplements were extra. I observed this healer "control" the minds of his patients for his own financial gain. Patients became dependent and obedient, unwilling to make any decisions without asking permission. They reported on fellow participants who did not adhere to the rules in a cult-like manner. One man who came into the center as a high-powered restaurateur was almost a vegetable after two weeks. His altered state was induced strictly by the acupuncture treatment and the fast he was on during his stay. This man became so passive that one Sunday morning when the fire alarm malfunctioned and went off repeatedly for twenty minutes, he could not even get up off the couch. When I suggested he take a walk and get away from the alarm, he began to theorize about the therapeutic benefits of this repetitious sound. He remained immobilized until the practitioner gave him permission to move.

It took me only this one experience to realize that as consumers, cancer patients are extremely vulnerable to being victims. This is something we must guard against. Making certain that our own welfare is placed ahead of the provider's priorities is one way to be reassured that we are getting what *we* need most. Having friends remain in contact when we go into a healing center helps us keep one foot in our everyday world. As it happened, it was this negative experience that pushed me out of the realm of the supposed spiritual healer and back into the conventional medical center.

The reentry was very difficult and I can see how it might deter many people who have tried to set their own recovery course. Most doctors were not very understanding or accepting of my previous decisions. One refused to treat me because I didn't do what she had recommended several months earlier. Other medical doctors felt the need to scold me or tell me that they would never have done what I did. The tendency toward a parent-child relationship was evident.

I knew I had to look ahead to live. It wouldn't do me any good to beat myself up about my previous decisions. Each decision was mine; I took responsibility for every one, knowing that I had made it with the best information available to me at the time. I didn't believe I could expect any more of myself than that.

My experience was that treatment alternatives can complement all types of therapy. Everyone needs to choose when to incorporate these alternatives; many resources are available to help us repair our battered systems. Conventional treatments treat symptoms and often have severe long-term side-effects. This is distinctly different from rehabilitating health to overcome a current condition and prevent future deterioration.

PART THREE:

Beyond Breast Cancer

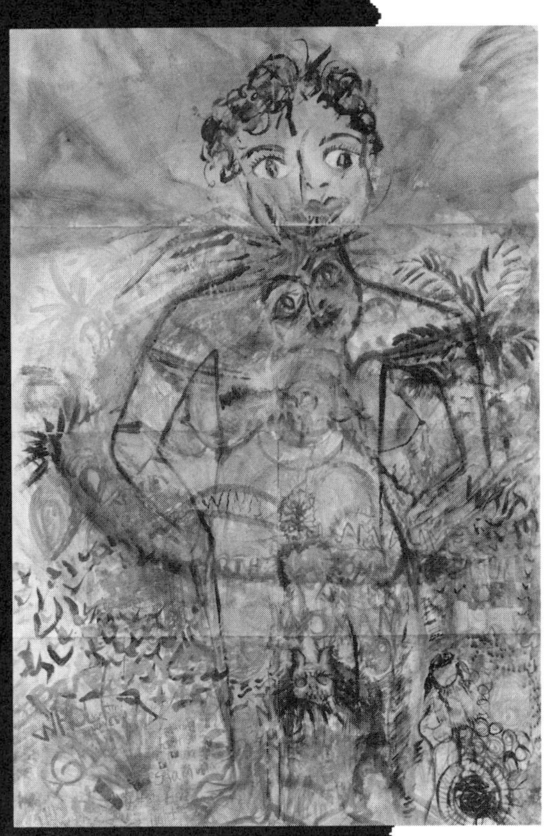

My Winged Breasts by Virginia Soffa

Ode to My Winged Breasts

This is my Goddess
She has winged breasts.
You can't see them,
but they're there.

I wanted to know
Where they were,
Where they went.

I found my lovely sweet
Young breasts
Right here beside me
On my quest.

Like two angels
They hover near me,
My two winged breasts.

During a workshop, Painting from the Source, *I discovered that I had a need to release my breasts, set them free and emerge as a new person. I am different today than I was for my first 40 years. I am flat chested, but I still feel whole. It's hard to explain. For two days I painted, I struggled with words and images. I delved into detail and painted more complexity than I ever have before. Then all of a sudden I grew another head and birthed out clearer about who I am.*

Passing through the anguish and turmoil, I broke through the top into clarity of vision, and set free my true spirit. I can paint more now, because I have painted what was inside, out.

My Winged Breasts
Virginia Soffa, Burlington, Vermont
Tempera on paper, 72½" x 48", 1994

8

Choosing Life

To be who we are, to acknowledge our personal purpose and place in the world, to live from our own truth is more fearful than exposing ourselves to the dark and the light which are intrinsic to nature and life.

Linda Marks, *Living with Vision*

A friend told me a story about a woman I'll call Hannah. Hannah was diagnosed with breast cancer when she was twenty-eight years old and married with two young children. After her two-centimeter malignant tumor was removed and it was determined that no lymph nodes were involved, she was reassured by her surgeon that she probably wouldn't need chemotherapy. Several weeks later, before she started radiation treatment, she visited the oncologist for a checkup. The oncologist delivered a grim verdict, telling her that if she didn't have chemotherapy immediately, she would have little hope for survival if her cancer were to recur.

Hannah was totally overwhelmed by this prediction. Fearful for her life, she rapidly consented to beginning chemotherapy in a few days. She refused to see another doctor, speak to other people, or consider any options.

My friend was shocked by the possibility that this doctor made a conscious decision to overload Hannah with this kind of threatening information so that she would be compliant. She felt frustrated that this young woman had closed the door on making her own choice about chemotherapy, and she feared what might result if Hannah proceeded with this treatment in this state of mind.

Dr. Joan Borysenko, in *Minding the Body, Mending the Mind,* shows that having a helpless or hopeless attitude about treatment works against the patient's healing process. She states, "Feeling constantly helpless can upset our endocrine balance, elevating the immunosuppressant hormone cortisol and destroying its natural diurnal [biological clock] rhythm. Chronic helplessness also depletes the brain of the vital neurotransmitter norepinephine, the chemical in our brains that is necessary for feelings of happiness and contentment."[1]

The most beneficial treatment for a woman who is being treated for breast cancer would be to encourage her to become an independent and self-actualizing thinker. Nonetheless, the whole national breast-cancer program revolves around perpetuating fear in women (as I describe in more detail in the next chapter, "Women's Rights in Health Care").

Women are misinformed, misled, and misunderstood when it comes to talking about their bodies. Many women have remained either naively or, perhaps, fearfully silent about their feelings about getting breast cancer; having their bodies mutilated; wearing heavy, warm, and poorly designed prostheses; undergoing dehumanizing, poorly substantiated drug and radiation treatments after surgery; being the subject of endless clinical trials; or not being taken seriously while being violated physically, spiritually, and emotionally by medical personnel.

Breast cancer evokes one of the greatest fears for women—a fear that is also experienced as paralyzing and silencing. Some women take care of their health problem with complete diligence—obeying the doctor's requests. Then they return to business as usual, happy to "get on" with their lives, wanting only to leave behind the fear and the memories of cancer because they want to believe they have "beat" it. When this happens, their motivations to change their diets, reduce work and family pressures, or stop smoking or drinking caffeine and alcohol are undermined and reduced to "do what the doctors say and you'll be fine." This kind of dogma neutralizes a woman's opportunity to really take control of her life.

I decided I wanted to deal with this one straight. I wanted to face the issue of death early; then I could get on with healing and living. Death was not something I feared—the pain of dying from cancer was what I feared much more. Realizing that I could take my own life to avoid the pain provided me with the control I wanted over my life and my dignity. It also worried me, however, because I had more reason to die than to live. I considered how, in death, I could be with my mother again. I could have the chance to accomplish in another life the things I had not accomplished in this life. Dying certainly can become an attractive alternative to a cancer patient. I knew I had to find a way to make my life meaningful so that death was not a convenient solution to what appeared to be unsolvable problems.

Some observers claim that women with breast cancer have different personalities than other cancer patients. I resented this whole concept, which smacks of blame, and I insisted that I didn't fit this profile. I wasn't compliant, in denial and repressing painful experiences, or habitually suppressing my anger. That's what I said and even believed. I could show anger; I rarely followed doctors' advice without questioning; and I saw a counselor regularly to discuss my painful experiences.

"I have always used my art as a way of reacting to or expressing what was happening in my life in my time in history. Breast cancer added a whole new dimension to my work: raw feelings, strong emotions. How fortunate I am to have this vehicle of expression, this way of getting my feelings out, this opportunity to share the message with others!"

Barbara L. Peterson
Indiana

Still, I wondered if there could be some validity to this concept. I hate to cry, I cower at the thought of expressing my anger by engaging in therapeutic screaming sessions, and I have submitted to medical procedures to prove I could, even when these procedures were not in my best interest. I rationalized that I was not perfect and that it was all right not to be perfect. What I missed seeing was my cleverness in masking my denial, pain, and anger. These feelings were old and deeply buried, and it would take an emotional breaking apart to free myself of this psychological baggage.

I remembered how my mother called my developing breasts "mosquito bites" when I was twelve years old. An elementary-school classmate pulled all her eyebrows and eyelashes out because her parents refused to buy her a bra. A high-school friend of mine put Band-Aids over her nipples because her mother told her she would be raped if boys saw her nipples erect. We all played with Barbie dolls that were too tall and thin and had pointy breasts. What impact did these events have on my self-image? Do women with breast cancer really have more issues around negative self-esteem than other women? Did we have more problems accepting our developing bodies? Did we get strange messages from family and peers about our breasts?

I resisted, I denied, and eventually I conceded that maybe I did fit the personality profile of a breast-cancer patient. It seemed as though once I admitted it, things began to change, and the change is still happening. I don't always feel good; yet I know emotional healing is also an essential part of my healing process. It wasn't enough to have medical treatment, change my diet, practice meditation and visualization, and take special herbs or drugs. None of these practices could override the emotional turmoil of discovering who I was, what I wanted, and what my limitations were.

Giving away our being is just a different kind of slow, numbing death. Embracing life, on the other hand, has to do with identifying our value to the world, seeing our purpose in life, learning to speak about what we see and feel. To me this meant becoming "real" and learning to accept my own set of scars and shortcomings, so that I don't have to pretend to be anyone else. My other life, my life before breast cancer, was like a performance where I was just one of the actresses. I played a part—the script had been given to me by my parents.

I had to set the record straight with my family, my friends, and the world. Then I could decide whether I wanted to continue in this life or to move out into another. The most difficult part of my healing effort, and a part that will continue for some time, has been becoming a new person—and finding a new way to live that fits my being.

Seeing and speaking the truth can lead to a lonely path. It opens the door to hurts and betrayals; it can feel like dying because of the enormity of the pain. The alternative is to forestall the pain by denying anything that we don't want to see. We can protect ourselves from this hurt, but at the same time we give up our inner being.

Carol S. Pearson describes the "warriors" among us as those who learn "to trust their own judgment about what is harmful and, perhaps most important . . . develop the courage to fight for what they want or believe in, even when doing so requires great risk—the loss of a job, a mate, friends, social regard, or even their very lives. . . . All the liberating truths, by themselves, fail! They fail partly because each is just part of the truth; all of us are like the proverbial blind men, each feeling one part and trying to describe a whole elephant.

"The hero ultimately learns . . . a *process.* The process begins with an awareness of suffering, then moves to telling the story and an acknowledgment to oneself and to others that something is painful. Then comes the identification of the cause of that pain and taking appropriate action to stop it."[2]

When I was diagnosed with cancer, I considered it a wake-up call about my life. I had a choice to make. Would I compromise myself and do what other people wanted me to do, as I had often done before? Or would I learn to speak with my own voice?

I told my story. I said publicly that I wasn't satisfied with the treatments that were being offered. When I discovered that breast cancer wasn't a curable disease, I said publicly that I felt betrayed. Such statements have been perceived as rocking the foundation on which breast cancer hope is built: "catch it early, trust your doctor, do what he says, and you will stand the best chance of being cured." I said publicly that I believed that treatments should be less harmful to the immune system. I asked that these kinds of treatment be examined.

Gloria Steinem, a breast-cancer survivor herself, says, "With breast cancer, especially, patients make the difference, not the physician."

Carlos Castaneda, in *The Teaching of Don Juan*, says, "Any path is only a path, and there is no affront, to oneself or to others, in dropping it if that is what your heart tells you. . . . Look at every path closely and deliberately. Try it as many times as you think necessary. Then ask yourself, and yourself alone, one question . . . Does this path have a heart? If it does, the path is good; if it doesn't it is of no use."[3]

The treatment path being offered today to women with breast cancer feels as though it is without heart—first because it attacks the body, and second because it creates a separation between the patient and the healing process. The patient becomes an object in need of repair, too helpless to participate in the repair process. Surgery, radiation, and chemotherapy are all alike in this respect: the patient sits or lies down passively while others act to repair the ailing body. The patient is passive, either being put to sleep or put into isolation to receive these treatments.

The relief comes when we are told no more cancer can be detected; yet this reprieve lasts only until the next test or some unusual pain occurs. Suddenly we realize we never are completely free of the possibility of more disease; we really can't be sure we have been cured.

As long as the cause of cancer is unknown and there is no certain way of preventing its return, many women understandably withdraw into denying that they have a chronic disease. For instance, during the 1992 silicone-implant debate, women testified that they wanted reconstruction so that they could get breast cancer "behind them," to go on with their lives. While it is admirable to move on with life and with a positive attitude, there are those who choose to forget and to do whatever it takes to make forgetting possible. I call this the "if I don't think about it, it won't come back" mentality. The patient is left alone, like a sitting duck, hoping that her number won't come up again. But the odds are against her, and somewhere deep inside, locked away behind her smile, she is aware of this.

Other women are horrified by what the disease has done to their body, and instead of expressing their anger and outrage, they withdraw into shame and embarrassment. They become unwilling to speak about it or look at it; they are ashamed that this could have happened to them. Like being raped, having breast cancer feels dirty, disgusting, humiliating, terrorizing. The breast-cancer image itself makes speaking about it repulsive to some people.

Some women who have undergone breast surgery volunteer their time to cancer organizations because so many who are newly diagnosed have no one to speak with. These volunteers willingly open their blouses so that newcomers can see for themselves that the results aren't so bad. Losing a breast or undergoing reconstruction can have visually acceptable results. Sometimes I have even thought *If more women could see what it looks like, maybe they wouldn't be so fearful.* Then I pull back from the quicksand notion of selling breast cancer as okay. I remind myself that it isn't all right—it's horrible, and I don't want to forget that. I can love my body the way it is, scars and all, because they remind me of what I have endured and of how strong I am. But I also want to find a way to ensure that other women won't have to have this experience to understand how important it is.

More than 1.6 million women previously diagnosed with breast cancer are alive today. Another million live with undetected breast cancer. Many women want to ignore the fact that these numbers represent an epidemic, and they bury their fears. Women survivor volunteers are taught how to assist other women in "accepting" treatment. Doctors want us, as patients, to be willing participants "for our own good." Volunteers are brought in to give testimonials that the doctors can't provide. Some women endure the "standard" treatments because they would be afraid to choose something else; they fear that no one would support them if they bucked the system. Since this is cancer, with a capital C, we believe we have only one choice. A common attitude is to just "get it over with soon" so the people around us don't have to endure *their* pain any longer than necessary. The tragedy is that if we agree to a treatment we aren't 100 percent sure of, then we are doing it for other people, not for ourselves.

Women who provide support can contribute to the problem of "stoic acceptance," if they are perceived as role models by new patients. Some are willing to talk about their experience, their treatment, their prognosis. Typically, a woman isn't accepted into the official American Cancer Society volunteer corps for breast-cancer survivors—Reach for Recovery—unless she has both conformed to standard medical treatments and "beat her cancer." If a woman's cancer returns, she can be removed from acting as a patient support volunteer. Although I suspect there are times when these volunteers talk about their dark side of breast cancer—their own fears, anger, and doubts—I have observed a high degree of optimism coming from this resource.

We are eager to celebrate survivorship, forgetting to honor the women who are lost. (Breast carcinoma in men accounts for 0.5% of all breast cancer in the United States.[4]) There are no holidays, no parades, no special cemeteries, and no songs to commemorate the tragedy of those who die of breast cancer. It was with this realization that I conceived of and created "The Face of Breast Cancer: A Photographic Essay," to be a tribute to women who died from breast cancer. Creating this traveling panel exhibition was my gift to the National Breast Cancer Coalition and to the families who have lost loved ones.

During and after a war it is the survivors who think about and talk about those who fell—their talent for cameraderie, their skill, and the manner in which they lost their lives. In the cancer battle, the survivors think and talk about themselves—their challenge, their courage, their success. They become role models for other survivors. Some act as though death must not be mentioned or else it might come true. An unfortunate outcome has become surviving, not living. The conclusion of breast cancer, however, is sadly similar for all women. The only difference is that for some it happens over a few years, and for others it takes decades. Most women with breast cancer ultimately die of the disease, no matter what their age, stage at diagnosis, or treatment.[5]

Still, each woman must attack the challenge believing that she will be the exception. We perpetuate this kind of thinking to get ourselves through the terror-producing treatment. If we can block our pain with denial we can surely survive. This is the dark side of cancer everyone fears most but talks about the least. Sharon Batt, a Canadian journalist and cancer survivor, in describing the NBC television broadcast "Destined to Live," relates an emerging perspective. Several women and one man spoke movingly on that program about their initial terror at the moment of diagnosis, but all had "conquered" their fear of cancer: "Pithy, bright messages dotted the testimonials," says Batt. "Everyone felt and looked great. . . . All had total faith in their doctors." But, she summarizes, something was missing. "Courage is all very well, but the picture was one-sided in the extreme. Patients who felt sick were not heard from, and those who have died were not acknowledged. Missing from the broadcast was any hint that the public should be concerned about breast cancer. The price of this Pollyanna stance is political impotence."[6]

Batt calls on breast-cancer victims to learn from AIDS sufferers. She describes women with breast cancer as appearing as "stoic optimists." "Women are encouraged to be hopeful about their chances, to press bravely ahead with their lives as if death were out of the question, and to choose among available treatments as if out shopping for a dress."

Although open discussion with fellow survivors is meant to help a woman to adjust to her new reality, survivor testimonials and support groups can also serve to push conformity and sell women on the idea that having breast cancer isn't so awful—"just look at all the survivors," is the implied message. As Batt observes, however, what these patients don't realize is how many other women *aren't* present. Support groups have proliferated especially since a 1990 study showed that women with advanced breast cancer had improved survival when they attended support-group meetings weekly.[7] Unfortunately, this research has been bastardized to support the formation of monthly, nonfacilitated groups, because most medical centers have yet to embrace or fund professional outreach and emotional support for breast-cancer patients. Perhaps the lack of motivation is that it doesn't make the center enough money.

Some volunteer caregivers become obsessed with the clinical guidelines and stereotype the unsuspecting newcomer. Asking patients their stage, the number of lymph nodes involved, or the size of their tumor seems innocent, but it is damaging when outsiders, family members, and untrained leaders misuse this information to quickly assess the newcomer's survival status. I think this evaluation system prejudices people's attitudes and can be very detrimental to women who are attempting to cope with an overwhelming amount of new information.

The most upsetting aspect about the way breast-cancer treatment is offered to the patient has a great deal to do with what is unspoken. Many women leave the doctor's office believing that after they go through the treatment, all they need to do is go back for their biannual or quarterly checkups. They believe that somehow their body will miraculously recover from the cancer and from the treatment, and their sole role as a patient in the whole process is to stay optimistic and cooperative.

When I entered the treatment "track," my body no longer felt like my own. Everyone else knew what was best for me. My biggest fear was the thought that a Reach for Recovery volunteer would visit me to say that I'd be all right because she was an example of a survivor. I didn't want to be told how "great" the treatments were or how I would look as though nothing had happened when I put on a wig or a prosthesis. I didn't want anyone to even imply that my life could be the same as before despite this disease or any of the paraphernalia that goes with it. What I did want, but got only from my psychotherapist, was someone to encourage my outrage, someone who was not afraid to hear that this disease had been handed down generation after generation, while women were silently resigning themselves to it.

In a May 1991 address "Who Cares? Women with Breast Cancer and Social Support," Dr. Patricia Bredenberg described research conducted in 1982 at Johns Hopkins Hospital: "Interviews of volunteers were conducted to determine how they viewed cancer patients: 60 percent said they would avoid persons with cancer; 81 percent said they would expect to be treated 'differently' as a result of cancer; 85 percent said they would themselves 'expect less' of a cancer patient—less general competence, less effectiveness at tasks, less assumption of authority."[8]

Bredenberg reported that her own patient interviews revealed that husbands often reacted to their wives' breast-cancer experience by closing the discussion with statements like "you had it; now it's over." And doctors trivialized the sometimes disturbing "phantom breast" sensations that occur after surgery. In essence, women are silenced by the very people they need to support their process of grieving and to help resolve their guilt, fears, and nightmares.

Explaining the importance of care in health-restoring programs for women with breast cancer, Bredenberg remarks, "Loss leaves metaphorical and mental as well as tangible scars. The challenge [for medical healers] is every bit as difficult as the surgery—and more, because the goal is not just survival, but living. It may take a year or two, but with c.a.r.e.—c equals communication, a equals assumption dumping, r equals respect , e equals education and empathy—most patients can rediscover not only the will to survive, but to live positively, to take pleasure in a world we rushed by before."[9]

To further demonstrate the value of support, Bredenberg cites a study in which it was observed that "men and women who predicted they would have adequate social network support (and were correct) at the time of diagnosis of cancer, lived longer than medically expected. Those who expected little support from friends and family (and were correct) died sooner than expected."[10]

The new cancer patient may dream that her illness will bring her family closer together, but cancer rarely seems to be a binding agent. My own experience was that this crisis, like other crises in my life, served to exaggerate the family's difficulties and our inability to support one another unconditionally. If I was going to find a reason to stay alive, I had to find it outside of my family unit. There were no children who relied on me, no parents left to worry about me. My sisters had their own concerns. Accepting this reality and finding my purpose was what ultimately gave me the strrength to choose to live. My realization came after a long process of looking at how I functioned in the world, how I led my life, and how I related to others. (For more about support systems, see Appendix 2, "A Message for Friends and Families of Women with Breast Cancer.")

One friend who was dying of her breast cancer decided that she wouldn't let her doctors decide when she should stop fighting. Although she had detected her breast cancer early, and she had submitted to all the recommended treatments—a bilateral mastectomy, chemotherapy, radiation, and eventually a bone-marrow transplant—her cancer was aggressive and kept returning. After the bone-marrow transplant, the doctors tried more radiation, but they warned her they had given her all there was and they had run out of options. They told her she had about three months to live. Being unwilling to give in to their death sentence, she decided to change her diet and develop a spiritual practice. She stopped eating processed foods filled with additives and preservatives. She stopped eating animal food. Instead of going to the hospital to die, she learned that her cancer was in remission; not a trace of the cancer could be found. Ultimately we all choose, either directly or indirectly, when we are willing to go. This woman also decided she wasn't going to let her doctors abandon her, even if they had exhausted their bag of cures.

As I offer this kind of anecdote, I fear that it may be read as blaming other women for not fighting hard enough, or as criticism of women who let go and decide death is easier. But my purpose in sharing this woman's experience is simply to illustrate the dramatic effect the mind and spirit have on our health, of the dramatic effect one little change might have or not have, depending on our underlying desire. All cancer decisions take courage. Understanding that any choice a woman makes is hers and hers alone is distinctly different from blaming someone for giving up too soon, or fighting too long, regardless of what family and friends might want her to do. This is not their decision. Freedom comes from believing we have the power to decide for ourselves.

A sense of paradox—between disease and health, bad and good, feelings of helplessness or feelings of hope—can be what undermines the determination of many women to fight to be well—to choose life—rather than fighting *against* the disease. We may want to know the truth about what we are facing, yet we can also admit that sometimes we are afraid to hear it. Life becomes a balance between reality and denial.

Going from a position of feeling helpless—helpless against the cancer, helpless about what to choose when none of the treatments have proved very effective, helpless to eat just the right foods and think just the right thoughts so we don't make matters worse, helpless to be the perfect patient—to the place of empowerment requires a shedding of many old ideas about how to create health.

Some women are reduced to being like children by their experience with breast cancer, others become warriors, and still others intellectualize about their experience. I have felt all these emotions myself at some time. I move in and out of different phases as if each is a part of my evolution to some other place, another stage, another life. I recognize that I am in the process of healing. I don't have answers, just more and more observations. I don't know where it will all lead—perhaps to death. But equally possible, it may lead me to life. I move forward knowing that part of the process is to keep making choices. Each day I have to examine what I am feeling and whether I am fulfilling my dreams. Each day I choose whether I will live my life openly or in retreat. Each day I choose whether I am going to think about breast cancer or ignore its existence. Both approaches seem to have value in my life. Mostly I choose to talk about it, but I also recognize the importance of having a life outside and beyond this experience.

Choosing life goes beyond deciding on a particular treatment. Choosing life has to do with breaking old habits, stepping out of the scripts that we have become accustomed to. It is not the end result that becomes critical to our success, but rather the process by which we arrive.

9

Women's Rights in Health Care

When there is no dignity, there is no strength.

Prisoner, Russian Gulag Firm 35

My own journey was initially about taking responsibility for my healing choices. But I soon learned that the issues surrounding breast-cancer treatment are feminist issues, intimately related to society's attitude about women.

GENDER BIAS AND WOMEN'S HEALTH

Women's health rights are in fact civil-rights issues: different rules have been applied to us because of our gender. Gender bias in health care is as systemic as breast cancer in a woman's body. It is a deeply ingrained reflection of American society that it is so prevalent it is often difficult to recognize.

Only recently have women organized around health-care rights in the same way they have united to fight for their freedoms around other issues. What constitutes acceptable health care for women being treated for female-dominant illnesses or for life-cycle changes that typically have been perceived as illnesses? Improvement in breast-cancer treatment has been impaired by our willingness simply to accept that what doctors have offered us is all that exists. Medical professionals are still trying to figure out how best to treat breast cancer so it won't recur, and they continue to use carcinogenic chemicals and therapies to cure women in the name of treatment.

Just because surgery, radiation, and chemotherapy are the only treatments offered at the local cancer center, it doesn't mean that they need to be accepted. Women submit to these life-threatening treatments because they believe there is no alternative. But as patients we are consumers, and we have enormous power if we can remain clear-minded and not become overwhelmed by the fear of dying. We can get better treatments. We can get better quality patient care. We deserve more than what is being offered today and what has been offered for the last hundred years.

Physicians often provide health-care information to women on a "need-to-know" basis. This approach to health care has traditionally kept women in a disadvantaged role: we aren't given all the facts about prescribed medications, we don't know enough about the subject to ask the necessary questions, and because our doctor is an "authority" we trust him ar her to do what's right, safe, and in our best interest. This form of control becomes essential to the patient-physician relationship. Every time a new situation occurs the patient must check with the doctor because the patient doesn't have enough knowledge to evaluate whether the event is minor or serious.

Women are the major consumers of medical care, yet the majority of the providers are male. Although the number of women attending medical school has increased enormously over the past fifty years, according to the Feminist Majority Fund,[1] female physicians haven't made major inroads into such fields as surgery and research. Women doctors are clustered in the lowest-paid specialties such as general practice, pediatrics, psychiatry, and internal medicine. In 1988 the American Medical Association released a report showing that female doctors earned 62.8 percent of the pay received by male doctors. Female student admissions may be increasing, but women still aren't moving into positions of power and authority. In 1991, none of the 127 medical schools in the United States had a female dean, and only 20.7 percent of medical-school faculty members were women. Women who have moved into positions of authority, like Dr. Bernadine Healy, former director of the National Institutes of Health, have done so at some cost. Forced to toe the administrative line (which opposed earmarking research dollars but has done so under the pressure of AIDS activists), she publicly recommended that the president of the United States veto any dollars earmarked for women's health research.[2] The threat, according to Healy, was that earmarked dollars would be destructive to the NIH. This is an example of a woman occupying a powerful position but unable to use her power to revamp the highly outdated, unworkable structure of the NIH.

This state of affairs in medical research and education is a microcosm of our educational system in general. Women make up the overwhelming majority of college students (76 percent), yet men (62 percent) and male thinking dominate the faculties of higher-education institutions. Teacher-education texts, for example, devote five times more space to men's accomplishments than to women's, despite the historical predominance of women in the teaching profession.

Women's voices are typically disregarded, and this is especially so when they express concerns about their own well-being. When a woman expresses a concern about a procedure, she is made to feel emotionally unstable. For example, our opinions about mammograms are invalidated by male and female professionals alike. If a woman complains that a mammogram hurts, she is told to think of the benefits—as though this will make it hurt less—while hearing the implication that the discomfort is all in her mind. Professionals devise programs to increase "patient cooperation" rather than respond to patient concerns by designing less assaultive procedures and equipment. Exploring the roots of gender-biased medical attitudes helps us understand why women's voices have been ignored. Even though women were humanity's early healers as medicine women, midwives, and caregivers, during the development of "medical science" in the last hundred years these early healers posed an economic threat to men who trained as physicians. Until the middle of the twentieth century, women had limited access to medical schools, which, according to Harvard biology professor and author Ruth Hubbard, were "operated by men for men."[3] Men of medicine were concerned that the profession might become "overpopulated, competitive (since modest upper-class women preferred to be treated by women), and economically threatening." These men held out beliefs that it would be "detrimental to women's health to be educated the same as men."

Reversing the tide of the increase in breast cancer in this country and internationally requires that we have a voice about our own health care. Knowledge is what is required to propel women forward. Knowledge provides us with the self-confidence we need to speak about our own experience. Because much of the expertise promoted in scientific and medical circles is gender-based, we need to actively review the basic principles that govern both the studies and the legislation.

The root of gender discrimination lies in our attitudes about what is "normal." Whatever women do or achieve is still gauged against a male standard of success. To gain credibility, women are expected to strive to measure up to preimposed male-established criteria, and conform to the male rules rather than being recognized for who they are. Yet, although aggressiveness is considered an asset to a businessman, for example, when a female professional is outwardly ambitious, both male and female colleagues may characterize her as a "barracuda" or, worse yet, a "bitch."

Ruth Hubbard points out that nineteenth-century scientists "proved" women's brains were inferior in size and capacity.[4] Although these theories were invalidated by the 1860s, the argument only changed from "Can women do it?" to "Is it good for them?" She describes the philosophy of Dr. Edward H. Clarke, chair of Materia Medica at Harvard Medical School, and author of *Sex in Education; or, A Fair Chance for the Girls*, published in 1874. Clark's book was a popular seller, going through seventeen editions. His philosophy—and what came to be the ideology of the times—was that women needed to avoid education because "women's physiology would be damaged if girls were educated the same as boys and therefore developed their brains rather than paying due regard to their menstrual function."[5]

Our hormonal function became the basis of discrimination that also fostered feelings of inadequacy in women. This attitude has been prevalent for generations, and it influences decision making, career advancement, and politics to this day. Women in business and professional fields, fearing career-advancement repercussions, plow through difficult days with PMS—or even breast-cancer treatment—fearful that any sign of weakness would confirm someone's underlying belief that women are less than adequate.[6] The language often used to describe women defines our actions in terms of our "moods" and results in stereotypes that say women are sex objects, contrary, emotionally weak, financially incompe-

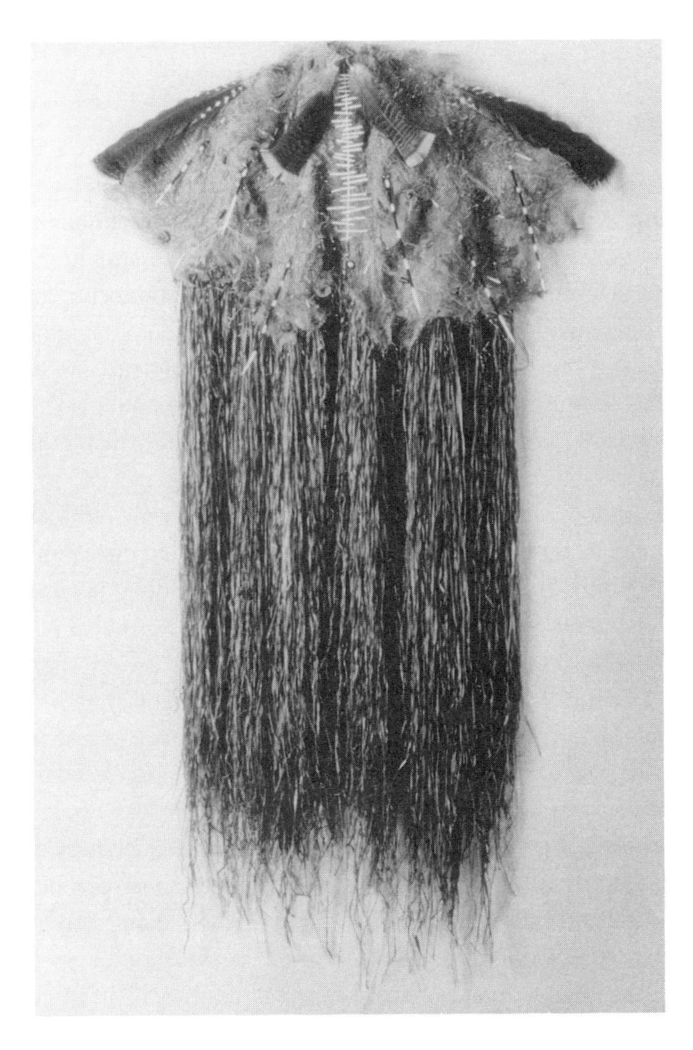

Warrior Woman
Cecelia Thorner, San Anselmo, California
Fiber, palm tree bark, raffia, quills, old beads, pods, copper wire, feathers, 50" x 33", 1992

"My experience with cancer left me feeling robbed of the power to affect my life before I even knew I had it. And yet, the sense of loss it created in me served as a catalyst for change, the spark that ignited my journey of self-realization. I wanted to take charge of my recovery and my life. I wanted to learn to recognize what my needs were and begin to take care of them. I wanted to uncover and explore passions and talents as yet undiscovered."

---

tent, and almost always hormone-influenced—that is, menstrual or menopausal.

Likewise, science has been used not only as a tool to explain the difference between the sexes but to "control" women, particularly our reproductive systems. Hubbard asserts that "science and technology always operate in somebody's interest and serve someone or some group of people. The pretense that science is objective, apolitical, and value-neutral is profoundly political because it obscures the political role science and technology play in underwriting the existing distribution of power in society."[7]

Rose Kushner, a pioneer breast-cancer activist, discovered this when she attempted to get the federal government to examine the safety of birth-control pills. She concludes, "After weeks of reading, telephoning, and interviewing to find out why we were not being warned about the dangers of the Pill, one short article gave me the answer—'economic incentive.' Economics and power often go hand in hand."[8]

The National Institutes of Health, the largest biomedical research facility in the world, is funded by the United States Congress with our tax dollars. Women represent 52 percent of the United States population, yet, in 1987, only 13.7 percent of the NIH budget was used to study women's health. Until 1991 (when Dr. Healy was appointed), there was no institute, center, or division, not even an office (the hierarchical categories used by NIH) for women. Women have been excluded from investigative research for treatment of diseases as common as heart disease primarily because of the threat experimental drugs might pose to an unborn fetus.[9] Scientists are concerned that a woman in such a study could become pregnant, or be pregnant, without realizing it, which would jeopardize both the study and the health of the fetus. Other people, both inside and outside the scientific community, contend that women's life cycles, menses, and menopause add additional complexity to study design.

ESTROGEN AND THE MENOPAUSE DEBATE

Characteristic of the medical approach to women's health care is the lack of scientific knowledge about women's natural hormonal functions. For instance, some theories regard menopause as an estrogen "deficiency disease" or an "endocrine disorder." This approach encourages prescriptions for hormone-replacement therapy (HRT) to correct the problems associated with such a deficiency. (While many women instinctivly resist taking hormones, their instinct is often overridden by scientific explanations that promote benefits.) HRT is hailed as a form of "immunization" against coronary heart disease and osteoporosis, but we hear little about how the risk of developing heart disease or osteoporosis compares with the risk of developing an estrogen-related cancer like breast cancer.

Menopause, not unlike breast cancer, is even treated as though it were a "new" disease because of increased life expectancy during the past one hundred years. Dr. Margaret Lock, writing in the *Lancet*, contends that "since the maximum life-span potential for a human being is estimated to be about ninety years and there is evidence that some people have lived to old age for at least one hundred thousand years, this argument is erroneous.[10] Nonetheless, cancer-causing, estrogen-based hormones are used to treat this so-called deficiency, and then after a breast cancer diagnosis she may be treated with more hormones, such as tamoxifen, to block cancer-producing estrogen.

Access to basic information about estrogen—how it interacts with our different systems, how our bodies utilize and discard excess estrogen—would be helpful to women. Instead, what we hear about are research "findings" that seem to blame women for their cancer and subtly reinforce gender-based stereotypes. One such finding publicly states an increased risk for breast cancer in women who do not have children before the age of thirty. Actually, studies document that breast-cancer risk is lowest in women who have children before the age of twenty, not thirty.[11] This information appears to demonstrate a physiological need for women to have children to decrease their risk of breast cancer, but in reporting the benchmark for increased risk as age thirty, science imposes society's standard that it is more acceptable for women to have families during their twenties rather than as teenagers. This advice about the timing of raising a family, as presented in association with breast-cancer risk, is in itself both simplistic and paternalistic.

Other scientists have suggested that breast-cancer risk is related to the number of menstrual cycles a women experiences in a lifetime. They have examined age at onset of menstruation and age at onset of menopause, in conjunction with the number of full-term pregnancies. The results of such research have been used to indicate a scientific argument for having big families to prevent breast cancer.[12] But the issue is in fact more generally rooted in the amount of estrogen a woman produces and utilizes in her lifetime. Methods of maintaining low estrogen levels have been identified as maintaining low body fat; getting daily exercise; minimizing the consumption of estrogen-loaded foods like chicken, meat, and milk; and avoiding estrogen-filled and estrogen-mimicking medications. There is evidence that these factors are especially important for teenagers and women in their twenties, who have developing breasts. Yet, because the evidence on risk factors is still inconclusive, no organization is encouraging this kind of "early prevention." Consequently, the available information on the relationship between hormones and breast cancer has provided no relief from the increasing incidence of the disease.

The menopause debate often points to psychological variables as well as somatic (biological) variables as the source of a woman's disturbances. An unspoken message that women "need fixing" to experience a normal life is demonstrated in the treatments offered. For many years doctors have encouraged an image of themselves as being our knights in shining armor who can rescue us from our own faulty hardware.

Psychosocial conflicts from earlier stages of the life cycle are also used to explain some menopause symptoms. These conflicts include the end of fertility, the death of one's parents, and "empty nest" losses. These times of transition, however, seem to be more of a problem for women in North America than elsewhere.

Margaret Lock[13] examined the cultural differences between 1316 women in Japan and 1310 women from Canada to illustrate the way menopause acts as a lightning rod for social and political issues. In Japan, the women surveyed associate *konenki* (menopause) with aging, and believe that "menopause is a gradual transition, which starts at forty to forty-five years of age and marks an entrance into the latter part of the life cycle. Graying hair, changes in eyesight, short-term memory loss, headaches, shoulder stiffness, dizziness, unspecified aches and pains, and lassitude are the signs most often associated with this transition. The end of menstruation represents only a small and relatively insignificant part of this process." Hot flashes and night sweats are less common for Japanese women. Of the Japanese women included in the study, 19.6 percent had at some time in the past had a hot flash, while the frequency was 64.6 percent in Canadian women.

"Distressing symptoms," associated with menopause in Western and European cultures, "are not usually linked in the Japanese mind to the lack of menses." Although women in Japan see gynecologists to deliver babies and terminate pregnancies, few seek help with menopausal symptoms. Only 4 percent of the women studied had been prescribed hormone-replacement therapy.

Japanese women are also less likely to use HRT as a prevention for heart disease or osteoporosis, because these are not high-risk problems for women in Japan. The political and social issues associated with menopause in Japan are different; for instance, the government applies pressure to keep middle-aged women out of the full-time work force. These women are encouraged to provide complete care of aged parents so that the government can deny the need for elderly-care facilities. Women who have "too much time on their hands" are more likely to run to the doctor with "insignificant complaints," according to Japanese ideology. Cultural socialization makes full-time employment for middle-aged women, elderly-care facilities, and menopause treatment economic luxuries.

THE PILL

Perhaps unique to Western culture, too, is that pregnancy and childbirth are considered to be more dangerous than the risks caused by increased estrogen. The 1969 FDA report on oral contraceptives detailed many adverse effects but declared the Pill "safe" in the report summary. Dr. Louis Hellman, the FDA committee chairman, was asked during the 1970 Senate hearings on this subject how he arrived at this conclusion. Hellman responded by saying that although the Pill presented some problems, it was "within the intent of the legislation." The Kefauver-Harris amendments that regulate the FDA say that determining drug safety involves balancing risks against benefits.

Hellman's recommendation included weighing the benefits of the use of the Pill in "curtailing population growth" against the risks of the Pill to women. In reports that assess the safety of oral contraceptives, pregnancy has also been identified as a condition that places women at risk. Like menopause, or even small breasts, pregnancy has been nebulously identified (by male standards) as a disease.[14]

The Pill introduced into the United States market in 1960 did not have to meet the rigors of long-term animal testing. Clinical trials were conducted for only three years before market saturation began.[15] Women who were in their late teens and early twenties in the 1960s now constitute the age group of women who are experiencing the greatest increase of breast-cancer mortality.[16] But the Pill, initially targeted to white, middle-class, college-educated women—the same group that is associated with the highest risk for breast cancer—experienced a shift in emphasis during the middle to late 1970s. As reports of harmful effects began to surface in the media between 1975 and 1978, use of the Pill fell by 25 percent.

The drug companies in turn sponsored their own studies and paid individual doctors to travel around the country to "restore patient confidence." General practitioners were encouraged by articles in peer journals to seek out patients and family planning clinics to make their services more accessible. These programs were designed to reach women who were less inclined to seek medical care, the "unmotivated" poor (as poor women who do not use birth control are described by the professionals), and women of color. Now breast cancer screening programs are targeted to these populations, which are experiencing greater incidence of, and mortality from, breast cancer.[17]

One researcher has estimated that more than one hundred million women have taken the Pill since it was introduced thirty years ago.[18] While the U.S. Agency for International Development, the federal department responsible for "population control," boasts that "over 60 million women around the world are now using oral contraceptives,"[19] some practitioners worry that many of these women still do not have the benefit of knowing all the risks associated with the Pill.

When I first started taking the Pill in 1969, there were no package inserts. Inserts used in the early 1970s made reference to animal studies, saying, "There is no proof at the present time that oral contraceptives can cause cancer in humans."[20] But even today, the information on package inserts describing all the substantiated risks is provided in small (seven-point) type on lightweight paper. The text is mostly technical and daunting to read. The contraindications continue to be downplayed by drug companies, by population-control advocates, and ultimately by the doctors who communicate these findings to their patients.

Both physician witnesses and pharmaceutical companies expressed resistance during the 1970 Senate hearings to including insert information, claiming that "vast numbers of women" do not have the ability or education to comprehend simple biological facts. Concerns about causing unnecessary "anxiety" in these women was offered as justification for not including written information. Rose Kushner describes a conversation in 1974 with a scientist at Roswell Park who maintained that many women would rather risk cancer than a pregnancy.[21] The "freedom of choice" premise behind this argument is similar to that used for both cigarettes and silicone implants.

Whether or not they recognize it, governments promoting oral-contraceptive use are actually party to a two-pronged method of population control, first by preventing pregnancy, and then—as it would appear from a global review of oral-contraceptive use, cancer incidence, and death rates—by contributing to the premature death of women (tables 5 and 6, page 172).

Although the Pill was introduced into Japan and Greece around 1968, it has not gained widespread acceptance in either of those places. Japan had only a 1 percent user rate and Greece 1.5 percent during the survey period 1970–1981. By contrast, the Netherlands had a 46 percent user rate, Belgium 37 percent, the United Kingdom (England and Wales) 28 percent as of 1976, Canada 27 percent, and the United States 23 percent.[22]

The American Cancer Society estimates that in the period 1984–1986, Japan ranked forty-seventh in breast-cancer deaths and Greece forty-fourth. The Netherlands, a country that experienced a rapid level of increased use, ranked sixth and Belgium seventh. The United Kingdom, Canada, and the United States instituted use of the Pill in the early 1960s while other countries watched. Most European countries had joined in by 1968.[23] Of the earliest users, the United Kingdom ranked first in breast-cancer deaths, Canada thirteenth, and the United States fifteenth (figure 4, page 173).

The United States, Canada, and Sweden (which ranks twenty-sixth in breast-cancer deaths) provide oral-contraceptive aid to underdeveloped countries. The United States is the largest provider and stands to benefit economically by the worldwide use of oral contraceptives, since the drug companies are located in the United States. According to the November 1988 *Population Reports*[24] of the sixty million women who use oral contraceptives, thirty-eight million live in developing countries.

TABLE 5

BREAST CANCER IN SEVERAL COUNTRIES: AGE-ADJUSTED DEATH RATES PER 100,000 POPULATION, 1984–1988

Country	Death rate
England & Wales	36.0
Scotland	34.0
Netherlands	32.4
Belgium	32.2
North Ireland	31.8
Canada	29.4
United States	27.4
Greece	17.9
Japan	6.7

Source of data: *World Health Statistics Annual,* 1984–1988[1]

TABLE 6

ANNUAL NUMBER OF BIRTH-RELATED OR METHOD-RELATED DEATHS ASSOCIATED WITH CONTROL OF FERTILITY PER 100,000 NON-STERILE WOMEN, BY FERTILITY CONTROL METHOD ACCORDING TO AGE

Method of Control and Outcome	15–19	20–24	25–29	30–34	35–39	40–44
No fertility control methods*	7.0	7.4	9.1	14.8	25.7	28.2
Oral contraceptives non-smoker†	0.3	0.5	0.9	1.9	13.8	31.6
Oral contraceptives smoker†	2.2	3.4	6.6	13.5	51.1	117.2
IUD†	0.8	0.8	1.0	1.0	1.4	1.4
Condom*	1.1	1.6	0.7	0.2	0.3	0.4
Diaphragm/ spermicide*	1.9	1.2	1.2	1.3	2.2	2.2
Periodic abstinence*	2.5	1.6	1.6	1.7	2.9	3.6

* Deaths are birth-related

† Deaths are method-related

Source: *Family Planning Perspectives* 15 (1983): 57–63.

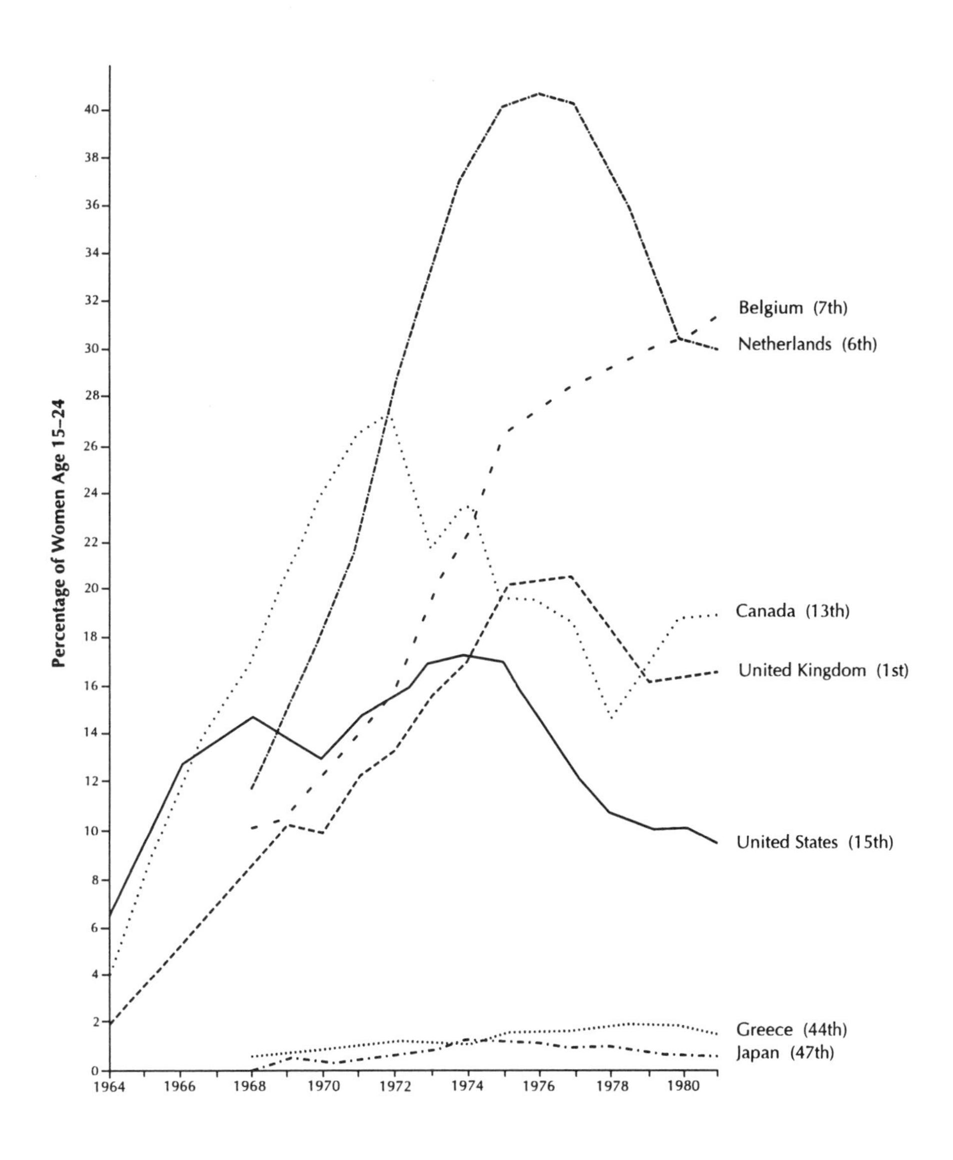

FIGURE 4

MINIMUM PERCENTAGE OF WOMEN AGE 15–44 SUPPLIED WITH ORAL CONTRACEPTIVES THROUGH COMMERCIAL CHANNELS IN SEVEN DEVELOPED COUNTRIES, 1964 TO 1981.

The number after each country's name shows its rank in breast cancer deaths during 1984 to 1986.

Women's reproductive and menstrual functions are therefore modified at the high cost of more than fifty potential health risks, several of which result in death. Women have been and are continuing to be given only limited verbal information about these risks, particularly the breast-cancer risks. Kushner attempted an early fight to restrict prescriptions for women who have a family history of breast cancer because of the possible dangers of the Pill. Yet even today these high-risk women are not limited in their use of oral contraceptives. Kushner reported that she was unable to find "a single scientist involved in breast-cancer research who believes OCs are safe where this disease is concerned. Everyone I queried was positive that adding large quantities of female hormones to a woman's body—especially a young woman's—is dangerous, regardless of the lack of statistical evidence."

Many studies show a clear relationship between oral contraceptives and increased breast-cancer risk. But what are we to think about a study that seems to have demonstrated that women who have taken the Pill and develop breast cancer have better survival rates?[25] Other studies also attempt to show the protective benefit of Pill use. We need to learn more about our own bodies so that we can apply our own common sense to this question and make a truly informed choice.

Reports on the safety of birth-control pills are so contradictory that even though I knew something about the existence of these reports, I continued to take the Pill. Now I can see that I dismissed this information because it was so confusing. When people are overwhelmed with conflicting information they have a tendency to disregard warnings. Complexity breeds helplessness and complacency. It becomes easier for people to brush off such reports with the conclusion, "Oh, everything causes cancer."

As it stands now, women's safety is bounced around the benefits-and-risk court as if our lives were just tennis balls. The Pill—the name, everything about it—is simple by design. Women are said to have been modernized by oral-contraceptive use. We are supposed to welcome the Pill as an opportunity for sexual freedom. Educated Women in the 1960s were convinced that the growing world population was a threat to our existence. The Pill was and still is marketed as the only genuine twentieth-century addition to family planning: It's new, it's for the benefit of the planet.

A glorified image of women who "have it all" is perpetuated daily along with this the-Pill-or-nothing mentality. My sister told me that her doctors and nurses treated her as though she were old-fashioned to use a condom for birth control after the birth of her first child. This raises another so-called benefit that comes with Pill use—the Pill releases men from birth-control responsibility. The use of the Pill, however, no longer negates the need for condoms, which provide some protection against transmission of HIV, the virus that causes AIDS, during sexual activity.

This "use the Pill" message reminds me of the kind of social pressure that was used in cigarette ads from the 1940s through the 1970s. Although drugs and medicine have been considered sacrosanct from the marketing gimmicks used by other product manufacturers, the *Los Angeles Times* reports that a study conducted at the University of California, Los Angeles—reviewing drug advertisements in leading medical journals—found that "advertisers frequently failed to balance information on a drug's effectiveness with information of its side effects and risks. Some ads studied, they suggest, could encourage inappropriate, even dangerous use of drugs."[26] The article goes on to say that "such ads are highly effective in encouraging physicians to prescribe the latest—and often most expensive—drugs." Not to anyone's surprise, the Pharmaceutical Manufacturers Association publicly objected to the study conclusions.

Once doctors are convinced of the wizardry of a particular drug, they exhibit the potential of becoming an extension of the drug-company sales team. Perks that consist of small gifts, free samples, and research grants seduce doctors, in subtle ways, to convey their confidence in the miraculous qualities of certain drugs and treatments. For instance, I was never warned about the Pill directly, and in fact I was one of the millions of women told by my respected doctor that it would *decrease* my risk of developing cancer: he assured me that there was a uterine-cancer-blocking advantage to taking the Pill, and he also reminded me that taking the Pill meant I had fewer premenstrual symptoms and no cramps. Oral contraceptives, unlike HRT or other hormone drugs, are considered "social medicine" because they are not primarily administered as a *cure* for anything. The Pill was the first drug ever distributed not for illness but as a prevention. (Preventive-drug marketing is now becoming more commonplace—an aspirin a day to prevent coronary heart disease, or tamoxifen to prevent breast cancer in high-risk groups.) Oral contraceptives, initially intended to be administered to healthy women, are now given to some not-so-healthy women as an all–around symptom regulator. I was one of these women.

In 1988, five months before my breast lump was detected, I went to my gynecologist and complained about irregular periods and low energy. He prescribed oral contraceptives to regulate my period. I was still taking birth-control pills the day my lump was diagnosed. When I told doctors I was on the Pill, none of them—including my gynecologist of ten years, who had prescribed the Pill—advised me to discontinue it at once, despite the dangers associated with this drug. The surgeon who did my biopsy said it probably didn't matter whether I continued taking the Pill, when I asked for his advice during my consultations both before and after the biopsy. Yet, the 1988 version of the package inserts for the brand of the Pill I was taking reads: "Contraindications: Oral contraceptives should not be used in women who currently have the following conditions . . . known or suspected carcinoma of the breast."

There is no way for me, or millions of other women, to undo all those years of taking the Pill. And today every woman who takes or has taken the Pill, is now eligible for one of the largest double-blind clinical trials ever instituted. Although the Pill industry has held up benefits that include everything from cancer prevention to sexual freedom, one nemesis to this industry remains the uncertain link to breast cancer. It is clear that the debate is far from settled and has not changed the way the Pill is prescribed. More disquieting evidence is published every year; yet the Pill is still distributed to teenagers and long-term users.

The increase in deaths caused by heart attacks is not statistically significant in women taking the Pill, yet if the Pill is in fact contributing to the increased incidence of breast cancer worldwide, we have a serious problem. In the United States, the FDA regulation process may cause people to be more suspicious of all drugs, and the federal dollars spent to promote their use in underdeveloped countries will also fall into question. Rising health costs have already become an emergency issue.

Transcripts of hearings held by the FDA on oral contraceptives and hormone-replacement therapy are costly and not easily accessible. But contained within this material, which stacks fourteen inches tall, is testimony from scientists and doctors about the lack of information available on dosage, frequency, and benefit-to-risk ratios for hormones.

Nonetheless, these drugs are prescribed daily, and estrogen-replacement therapy (ERT) has been in use for more than forty years.[27] Unlike implants, about which little research existed at all, so much information about estrogen exists, and so much of it is contradictory, that a woman would require a career in estrogen analysis to draw any personal conclusions. Women who take drugs or use medical devices often hold the assumption that these treatments and medications have been researched thoroughly enough to be verified by some authority as safe. We are now becoming more aware that this isn't always the case. "Safety" continues to be a subjective concept in medicine, and when deciding about such drugs, most individuals—whether doctors or patients—have to rely on the information provided by the manufacturers rather than wade through the mounds of research available on this topic.

Women who accept experimental treatments, and pay dearly with their bodies and financial resources, do so because they think they must to survive. I hear over and over again, "What choice do I have? If I want to live I have to take this treatment."

Alisa Solomon views this problem from a feminist perspective in the *Village Voice* in 1991.

> When it comes to diseases that attack women, an additional set of issues makes medicine political. With rape and battering on the rise, the assault on reproductive rights continuing to escalate, and little real change from the culture of woman-as-ornamental-object, women in America are still not granted dominion over their own bodies.[28]

A comparison with battered women may be illuminating. A report presented at the American Psychological Association's 1991 conference in San Francisco related that "battered women who stick by abusive men are not crazy—like hostages, they are trying to survive a potentially deadly situation."[29] Might this same psychology apply to women with breast cancer? The fear of death can create a unique bond between the patient and her doctor. Abusive behavior begins with the doctors' expectation that women with breast cancer should relinquish to "the experts" control of their bodies, their power to make decisions, and their will to choose what's right for them. For many women, it is difficult if not impossible to stand up to their doctors. Their doctors are their saviors—why should they oppose them? Fear of losing a lifeline—the family

FIGURE 5
CANCER STATISTICS, 1991

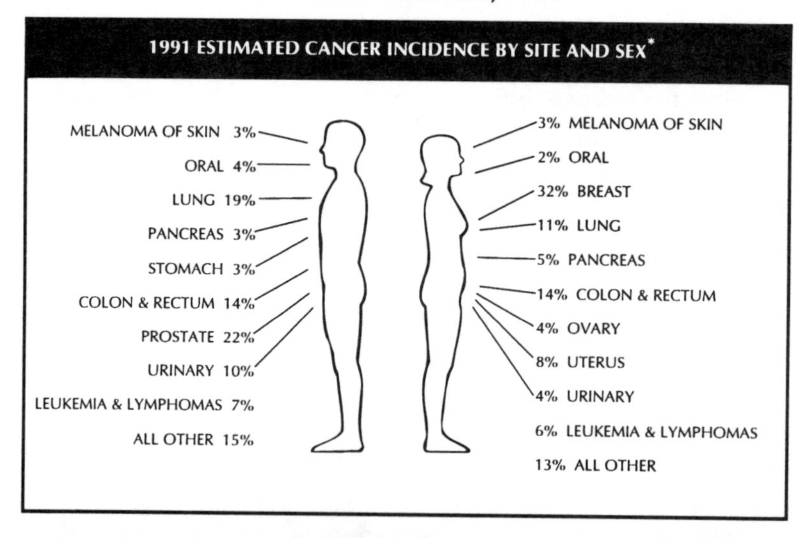

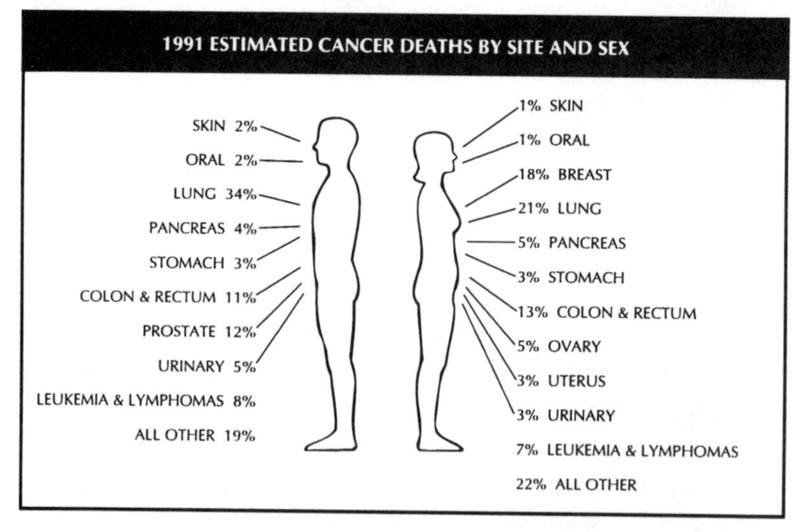

* The estimates of the incidence of cancer are based on data from the National Cancer Institute's Surveillance, Epidemiology, and End Results (SEER) program. Nonmelanoma skin cancer and carcinoma in situ have not been included in the statistics. The incidence of basal and sequamous cell skin cancer is estimated to be more than 600,000 in 1991. Mortality statistics are based on deaths reported to the National Center for Health Statistics, U.S. Department of Health and Human Services. Mortality rates are age-adjusted to the 1970 U.S. population.

member, friend, or doctor—is what keeps many women from speaking their minds about what they really want.

Breasts, although a part of the reproductive system, often seem to be treated as dismembered objects. Historically, bulbous breasts were ritualized in association with the fertility goddess—nurturing, life giving, and earth-connected. Now they seem to be the designated sex symbol of the twentieth century. Our relationship to this part of our bodies has become defined by the fashion industry, while others are satisfied to accept breast cancer as an all-time mystery. Perhaps it's time to reconnect with how our breasts are a virtual part of creation and its evolution.

Breast-cancer incidence exceeds that of all other types of cancer by 10 percent (figure 5). Is breast cancer a feminist issue? Is it a political issue? Can women continue taking the Pill, HRT, or DES while this debate—which isn't really a debate, but a marketing problem—continues? Women need to be taught that one study doesn't nullify another just because it shows inconclusive results. As long as the results remain in question, women will need to assess and determine their own risks. We need to protect our sisters, daughters, and friends. We no longer can rely on our government agencies, with their entrenched economic agendas, to protect us from profit-hungry industries.

Women's health has not been the priority of science for centuries. Instead, we have been used to test out medications, used as tools for increasing or decreasing population growth, and now used as a source of profit for health-care providers. Until the abuse of women's health-care rights ends, women will have to set their own standards; boycott products that have unresolved safety concerns; demand improved, less dangerous, and less abusive diagnostic and treatment options; and make known the kind of care we want.

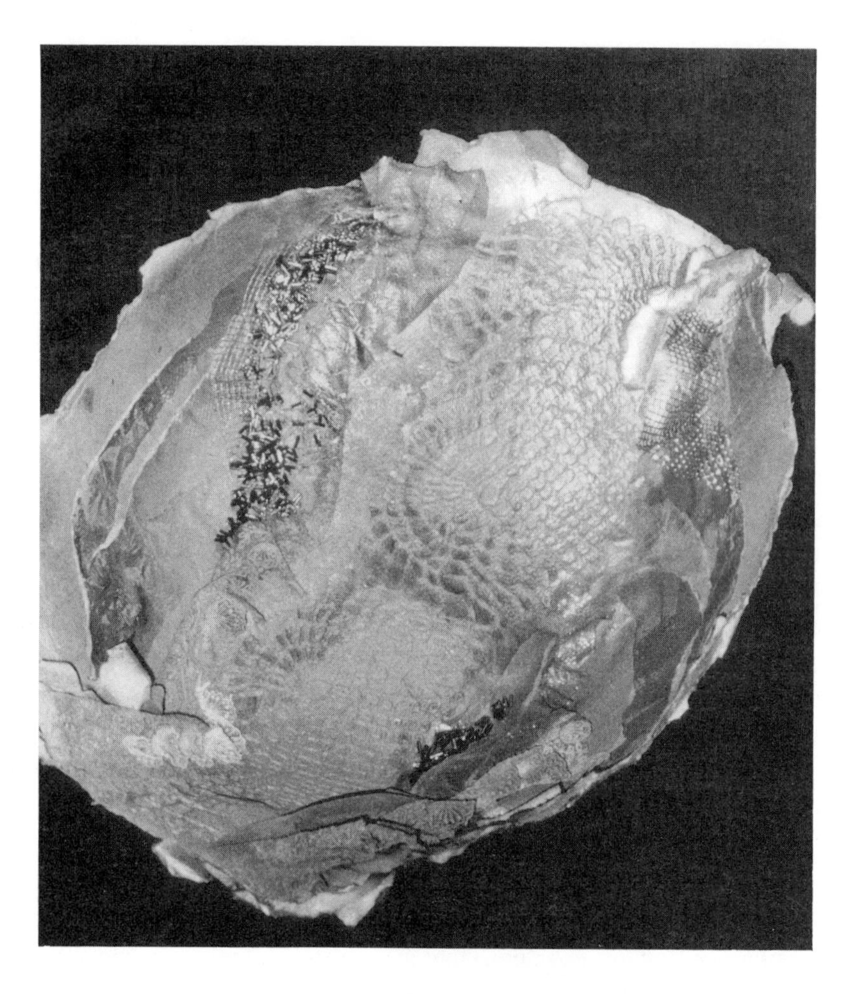

Sisters
Marcia Rhodes, Richmond, Vermont
Handmade paper with collage elements, 11" x 18" x 17", 1993

"As I witnessed [this] container taking shape in my hands I had a growing awareness of my own physical presence as a vessel and form-holder in this lifetime, which inspired me to recognize the significance of my actions and their effects on future generations."

10

The Politics of Breast Cancer

"In the '70s and '80s, we learned that the personal is political. In the '90s, the world must learn: the political is personal.

Gloria Steinem, *Revolution from Within: A Book of Self-Esteem*

It is easy to make a case for breast cancer as a personal disease—the scars and changes it leaves are physical, psychological, and spiritual. Breast cancer appears to be attributed to causes that are quite personal: our genes, what we eat, the drugs we take, environmental exposures, the way we cope with stress, our self-esteem, perhaps even our karma. The treatments for breast cancer are personal; they change our bodies, our sexuality, our lives. People might feel sorry for a woman with breast cancer, but most want breast cancer to stay *personal*—the problem of the person who gets it.

I believe the time has come to share the problem of breast cancer with everyone who isn't getting it. Many people don't know that *six times* more American women died from breast cancer during the Vietnam war years than all the Americans who died as a direct result of that war. Many people don't realize that testing and expensive screening programs are not prevention, nor have these approaches noticeably improved incidence or mortality trends. Our leading scientific research center, the National Cancer Institute (NCI), denies that breast cancer is affecting more younger women. It says that it has made great strides in treatment and that a cure is "just around the corner." The people who set up programs and who direct research include the National Cancer Institute, the National Institutes of Health, and the Centers for Disease Control, all funded by the United States government with our tax dollars. Until the 1993 federal budget was passed, none of the cancer research dollars was "earmarked" for breast cancer study.

Breast cancer is a political disease. The direction health policy takes results from numerous factors, including the party of the president. In 1992, during the Bush-Quayle Administration, the vice president set up a special commision on breast cancer to make recommendations about how breast cancer is currently treated—what we know and what we need to learn. The members of this commission were all political appointees. How a particular disease is funded is very political. Does it benefit the legislator to support this cause? The fact that breast cancer is non-partisan has its benefits; nonetheless, politics intervenes in philosophy when the sources of research funding—federal dollars vs. private dollars—are determined. To which agencies these funds go is also political. Most government agencies are territorial about programs, capital improvements, and staffing because they are all competing for the same funds. At present the government has no comprehensive plan to coordinate agency research or services. However, activists are pushing for this kind of effort, which would include patient representation. Because breast cancer is a "money-maker," women become victims of both the disease and the organizations that benefit from its continued existence. For instance, aggressive screening programs and state-mandated mammography-access programs that cover screening costs may well indicate a vested interest in bringing more women into a one-way process of detection and treatment even though we know that breast cancer cannot be prevented by screening.

Breast cancer is also a social disease. It is a "woman's disease" that has remained without a known cause or cure for longer than any other disease. It is a disease of neglect, abuse, punishment, guilt, and control. The neglect is evident in the lack of progress in finding causes and preventatives and a tendency to remain in a mode of treating the symptoms rather than the whole body. Abuse is evident in the procedures used daily for detection and treatment. A punishing attitude blames women who are childless, overweight, over fifty, depressed, or who openly share the consequences of their disease. I remember watching a network television news report on magnetic resonance imaging (MRI) technology for detection of breast cancer, in which the anchorman participated in this blaming of women with the statement: "Women die every day because they did not get a mammogram soon enough." (The AIDS movement has a slogan for this: "Fight AIDS, not people with AIDS." With breast cancer, as with AIDS, the separation between the person and the disease becomes lost in the way disease is diagnosed and treated.) Guilt occurs because society tells a woman that she is less of a woman without perfect breasts, that she is a personal failure for getting breast cancer. Guilt causes women to feel embarrassed and to seek invisibility about their experience with breast cancer. Embarrassment is a powerful emotion. It contributes to denial, false optimism, and immmobility. Women are being controlled by the threat of breast cancer, and this control is dependent on fear. The disease creates an increased usage of medical services and inspires unquestioning cooperation, instilling dependency on the medical system to provide answers, and exhausting our financial resources and our energy, thereby rendering women powerless over their own bodies.

Embarrassment has paralyzed progress in treatment because even women in the scientific community remain quiet. As long as women with breast cancer accept what is available and don't expect better, scientists are not motivated to investigate more creative, less mutilating diagnostic methods and treatments. Finding the cancer earlier isn't good enough. The emphasis needs to be placed on restoring health and eliminating breast cancer. But years of early-detection publicity have only blurred the distinction between detection and prevention and created a false sense of assurance that breast cancer is curable, suggesting that providers and patients have different motives.

Breast cancer is one result of our neglect of women and their health. Until recently we have simply accepted the outcome of the breast cancer epidemic, year after year witnessing more and more women being diagnosed and then dying. As long as the causes are treated as irrelevant, the problem will continue, because breast cancer will remain a mystery.

Overwhelming evidence shows us that the chemicals and preservatives used to increase crop production and extend the shelf life of foods are carcinogenic. The rise in breast-cancer incidence may be an indication that these substances are used at the expense of women. Women's bodies may be more sensitive than men's to added hormones and chemicals. A few small studies have demonstrated that women with breast cancer have higher levels of certain chemicals in their breast tissue. Women in a Connecticut study had higher levels of PCBs and p,p'-DDE (a breakdown of DDT); women in a Finnish study were observed to have higher concentrations of beta-hexachlorocyclohexane (b-HCH) in their breast fat. "Levels of lindane, dieldrin, and heptaclor epoxide were also elevated in the tissues of cancer cases compared to controls,"[1] but results did not reach a statistically significant level. Thanks to politics we don't have any solid answers, since women remain underrepresented in large-scale, federally funded research studies.

Looking beyond our personal situations—what's available at the local hospital, and whether insurance covers expenses—is difficult but necessary if this rising trend is going to be reversed. Women from the baby-boom generation who get breast cancer have started to do more than ask for options. They are trying to become informed consumers, and they are starting to look at the subtle but pervasive sexism that exists in funding, research-study design, and treatment.

When I started my own investigation into breast cancer, I couldn't believe that sexism would be at the root of this issue. I frequently heard people say, "If breast cancer were a male disease, it would already be preventable." Now I have seen for myself that sexism is part of the reason breast cancer has been ignored as a health issue and exploited as a political and economic issue.

MAMMOGRAPHY SCREENING IS POLITICS, NOT PREVENTION

As breast-cancer incidence figures have increased, scientists have attempted to explain the rise. (See table 7, page 185.) The NCI believes that only part of this increase can be attributed to more frequent detection as a result of increased screening. Carcinoma *in situ* tumors, however, are not included in American Cancer Society statistics or in the data bank for the NCI, known as SEER (Surveillance Epidemiology and End Results). A greater number of these smaller cancers (80 percent) are being diagnosed by mammography, yet until 1993 the NCI had no means of getting an accurate count. So far, the actual number of women undergoing cancer treatment is not available. Breast-cancer incidence is likely to be much worse than anyone wants to admit.

TABLE 7

BREAST CANCER INCIDENCE IN THE UNITED STATES

1991* Report	Incidence/100,000	1994* Report	Incidence/100,000
1973	83.9	1973	82.4
1974	95.9	1974	94.5
1975	89.0	1975	87.7
1976	87.0	1976	85.2
1977	85.3	1977	83.8
1978	85.6	1978	83.9
1979	86.6	1979	85.3
1980	86.8	1980	85.0
1981	90.8	1981	88.5
1982	91.2	1982	89.0
1983	95.2	1983	83.0
1984	99.6	1984	96.6
1985	106.1	1985	103.4
1986	108.5	1986	106.0
1987	116.5	1987	112.3
1988	112.9	1988	109.6
		1989	105.5
		1990	108.8

* Statistical reporting has a three year lag time; age-adjusted to 1970 population.

Source: Reported by the National Cancer Institute's SEER (Surveillance Epidemiology End Results) program

In attempting to update the previously reported incidence I discovered that the latest version is limited to "invasive" breast cancer and therefore reflects a slight decline in incidence.

That breast cancer kills only women who wait, and that breast cancer is dangerous only if neglected, are widely held assumptions. The women who have the disease are in essence blamed for not being somehow more responsible, more vigilant. Yet early detection is now known not to be "early" at all; a cancer detectable with mammography is approximately six to eight years old. Women are repeatedly urged through public health programs to get a mammogram without being told that this test has limitations and is not even suitable for women of all ages. Detection through screening is being confused in the popular press with prevention, and the American Cancer Society (ACS) and other breast cancer prevention programs do little to dispel this myth. Early detection seems to provide some women who have cancer with some additional lead time, but it is still uncertain whether long-term survival is improved in younger women.

Increasing awareness about breast-cancer screening also has the potential to increase awareness about the need for charitable donations. "Look at all we are doing," the organization is able to say. "We are providing an important service by promoting prevention." But even though one organization—the ACS—has a high profile in promoting screening awareness, it has no special fund for breast-cancer research. In fact, one woman shared her story at a Mother's Day rally in Vermont sponsored by the Breast Cancer Action Group: This woman had lost her sister, cousin, and mother to breast cancer. Most recently, when her mother died, the family decided to make a significant contribution to the American Cancer Society for researching breast cancer. Four days after her mother's death, the ACS called from Washington to say the family's donation could not be accepted if it was "earmarked for breast cancer." The family was devastated and withdrew its contribution.

Breast cancer is a socially "promotable" disease. Numerous organizations "race for the cure" and rally for funds, all the while directing the majority of these dollars into programs that push screening and private research. First we were told we needed bigger and better facilities. This created a need for greater usage and more participation. Now scientists are recommending that they need better images and technical training. They say screening will be able to do the job; it will save lives if we can meet a "gold standard" of quality. The professionals keep telling us how they've made the film better, the radiation lower, the compression better. The technology has improved, but the ratio of women dying has not. One out of four women will die; this has been the ratio for over thirty years.

Despite the promise made by some of the big cancer organizations, early detection has proved to help only 30 percent of the women diagnosed. If you happen to be one of those women, mammography seems like a lifesaver. If you happen to be part of the 70 percent, mammography screening is a betrayal, because you are given false assurances that nothing is there when in fact you have breast cancer. Still the statistics are conflicting. Some studies say eventually mortality will be improved. Others say screening will not improve mortality and may even increase deaths of women younger than fifty by giving a false sense of security when they get a negative report. Screening has been in use for more than twenty years. Yet while incidence has increased, mortality has remained at the same dismal level for sixty years. Until this ratio changes, scientists will continue to have a difficult time making a case for improved mortality resulting from early detection.

The ACS sponsored a massive study to demonstrate the benefits of breast-cancer screening. The Breast Cancer Detection and Demonstration Project (BCDDP), as it is officially called, selected 280,000 women and conducted a nonrandomized uncontrolled study. Because of its magnitude, this study is often cited when experts want to show that early detection reduces mortality, even though the study does not meet the research gold standard of being controlled and randomized. The claims that early-detected breast cancer is 95 to 100 percent curable nonetheless come from this study.

Contradictorily, both NCI and ACS scientists otherwise caution against using nonrandomized uncontrolled studies as a basis for early-detection programs. For example, with regard to early detection for lung cancer, scientists have stated that a screening program is not warranted. "To recommend an annual chest x-ray or sputum cytology would violate one of [the ACS's] main concerns: that there must be good evidence that each test or procedure recommended is medically effective in reducing morbidity or mortality."[2]

According to the ACS, the evidence for the effectiveness of a good screening program would include the following criteria:

1. An understanding of the natural history of the disease
2. Easy detection of tumors in an early and highly curable stage
3. An effect on death rates and incidence that warrants the costs and the risks
4. The ability to detect cancers in an asymptomatic population

For instance, the Pap smear detects cervical cancer in a precancerous phase, which is highly curable. This screening test has achieved a steady decline in mortality during the past fifty years. It is a successful early-

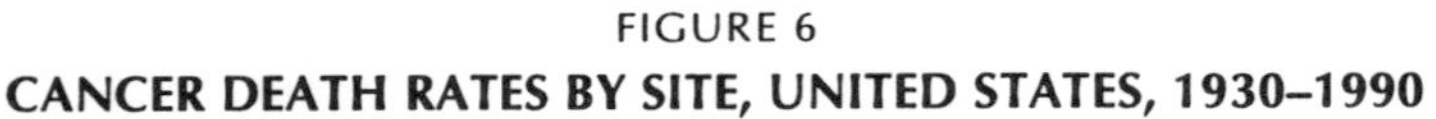

FIGURE 6

CANCER DEATH RATES BY SITE, UNITED STATES, 1930–1990

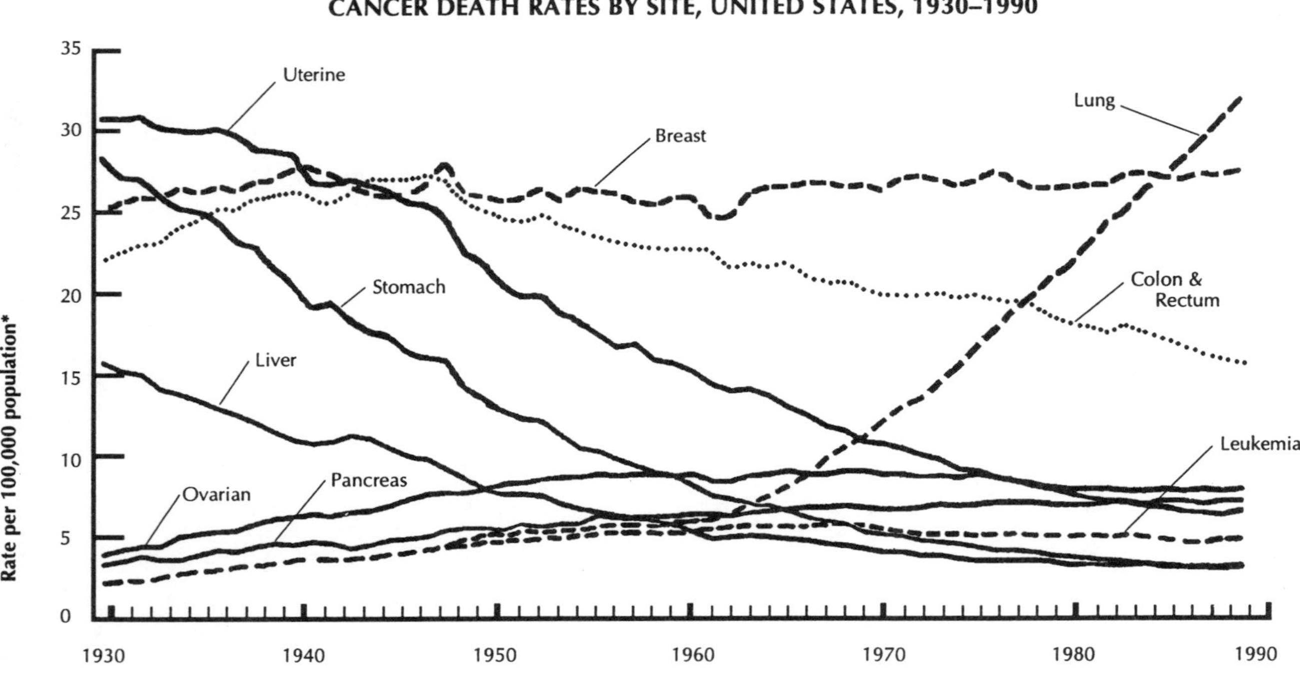

* Rates are per 100,000 and are age-adjusted to the 1970 U.S. census population.

Source: American Cancer Society, *Cancer Facts and Figures 1994.*
Source of data: National Center for Health Statistics and Bureau of the Census, United States.

detection program that saves the cost of more expensive later interventions, in addition to saving lives. Although this particular test requires an annual office visit, a compromising exam, and sometimes medical follow-up, women have complied, recognizing the benefit.

On the other hand, although a blood test has been developed for screening for ovarian cancer, the CA125 is far from routine. Likewise, the chest x-ray to screen the high-risk smoking population for lung cancer would not be effective because doctors are not able to provide a "standard cure" and they do not understand the "natural histology" of these cancers. In the case of lung cancer, "failure to observe any improvement in survival in those who accepted screening is evidence that there was no effect."[3]

Mammography screening meets only one of the above ACS-specified criteria: the test can detect cancers in asymptomatic women. Many researchers have tried to demonstrate that the cost, risks, and effect on death rates and incidence warrant screening, but their findings have been inconclusive, and screening ultimately has not caused a downward trend in either incidence or death rates. Several studies demonstrate that there is no conclusive evidence to support mass screening of women under fifty, yet federal and private funds support programs for screening all women over age forty—in some circles, thirty-five.

In fact, a research debate arose in 1991 when the London *Sunday Times* reported on results from the Canadian National Breast Screening Study (NBSS), the largest study of women under fifty ever carried out anywhere in the world. Fifty thousand women aged forty to forty-nine were studied for eight years. The study results indicated that screening mammography may have only a minimal effect on lowering death rates in women over fifty, and it may also be related to an *increase* in death rates in women under fifty.[4] One explanation offered for this statistical result is that there is an indeterminate number of false negative readings, which give women and their doctors a false sense of security, thus causing a delay in detecting the cancer. The *Journal of the American Medical Association* reported in April 1990 that 30.7 percent of the patients studied in Australia have false negative results, and these were "more likely to be obtained in younger women."[5] Professor Anthony Miller, director of the Canadian study, told the *Sunday Times* that the results also suggested that one reason for the increase in deaths was the failure of conventional cancer treatment for younger women. "Screening only works in the context of having good treatment," he concluded. This study has come under attack for not using the same equipment at all sites. However, this circumstance accurately reflects the variables most women encounter at screening centers. The authors of the NBSS claimed that the information in the London *Sunday Times* was not released with the study author's permission and needed further review. Subsequently this review was conducted, and the results as stated have been confirmed.

Studies in several countries have shown varying increases in deaths of women under fifty following the launching of aggressive screening programs.[6] In Britain, national screening is not advocated for women under fifty.

According to Petr Skrabanek of Trinity College, at the University of Dublin, Ireland, the "Health Insurance Plan" (HIP) study—the first study to show promise for mammography screening—had missed "40 percent of breast cancers [with] mammography."[7] A United States General Accounting Office report to Congress in January 1990 stated that 29 percent of the mammography facilities applying for accreditation did not meet American College of Radiology accreditation standards. The reasons for failure included poor clinical image quality (36 percent), poor phantom image (a dummy breast with hidden particles) quality (36 percent), and excess radiation dose (3 percent).[8]

Most women are unaware of the radiation levels in mammography. Mammography radiation is measured as mean glandular dose: the dose at the center of the breast. The American College of Radiology standards allow up to four hundred millirads (mr) per view.[9] This level is determined by using a phantom to simulate a breast. When I surveyed eighteen facilities to compare radiation levels, the radiologists themselves didn't know how their facilities compared to others (table 8).

I have been told that radiation levels are not discussed with patients because no one wants to say anything that might discourage women from getting their annual mammogram. This is the area in which I have seen the most effort to silence criticism. I have heard from a variety of sources, "We don't want to do anything to deter women after we have worked so hard to get cooperation and compliance." If this is the case, would organized medicine really be willing to replace the mammogram with a blood test if a tumor marker were developed? These comments are made

TABLE 8

VERMONT MAMMOGRAPHY FACILITY SURVEY SUMMARY

Facility	Accredited	Millirads[1]	Comments[2]
Aesculapius Medical Center	Yes, since 1991	57mr	
Brattleboro Memorial Hosp.	Yes, since 1989	60 mr	
Rockingham Memorial Hosp.	No longer doing mammograms		
University Health Center	Yes, since 1988	87 mr	
Copley Hospital	No*	90 mr	
Springfield Hospital	Yes	91 mr	
North Country Hospital	Yes, since 1990	95 mr	
Fanny Allen Hospital	Yes, since 1988	99 mr	Dedicated processor
Central Vermont Medical Ctr.	Yes, since 1989	100 mr	Dedicated processor
Porter Medical Center	No*	117 mr	
Vermont Radiologists	Yes	118 mr	Dedicated processor
Rutland Regional Medical Ctr.	Yes, since 1967	125 mr	Has 2nd unit
Mt. Ascutney Hospital	No*	150 mr	
Gifford Medical Center	Yes	165 mr	
Northwestern Vt. Regional Hosp.	Yes, 1994	165 mr	
Southwestern Vt. Medical Hosp.	Yes, since 1987	190 mr	
	2nd unit	204 mr	
Northeastern Vt. Regional Hosp.	Yes	212 mr	
Convenient Medical Care	No longer doing mammograms		

[1] Single-view mammogram, mean-glandular-dose for a breast phantom with grid

[2] All facilities reported having dedicated mammography units

* In process of applying

Survey conducted for *Hospital News,* January 1991; accreditation status updated in 1994.

Sept. 1991 update: A statewide report has just been completed by the State of Vermont Department of Occupational and Radiological Health and is being reviewed by the State Commissioner of Health. This study includes FDA screening capability analysis figures. Early remarks by study director and Senior Health Physicist Paul Clemons are that there was "not very much difference in quality or radiation levels between accredited and non-accredited facilities." Balance of dose and image quality became final determinating factors. No facility in Vermont scored below minimum quality levels.

with the highest of intentions even by women health practitioners who forget that they are withholding the very information women need to make an informed decision. Since the ACR does not impose a limit on the number of views that may be taken during any one visit, it is up to the patient to understand that a "consumer beware" warning is entirely appropriate.

In *Radiation Protection: A Guide for Scientists and Physicians,* Jacob Shapiro maintains that "retakes because of faulty films [of all types] were said to be responsible for about 27 million additional films per year. . . . Defensive x-rays, a consequence of the malpractice mores of the era, comprised a significant percentage of the 271 million examinations per year."[10]

As the studies previously described in "Searching for the Cause" demonstrate, considerable evidence exists to indicate that ionizing radiation has a strong causal relationship to increased cancer risk. Radiation is cumulative in our bodies. Mammograms present one of the higher levels of diagnostic radiation. Still, no one is keeping track of our individual radiation exposure. The mean-glandular-dose is only an average and does not actually represent the amount of radiation each person will get. Radiation dose depends on size and density of a woman's breast as well as on the equipment used for exposing and developing films, the type of film used, whether a grid is used, and the amount of compression. Grid use can vary depending on the size of a woman's breasts. Radiation exposure risks have a long latency period.

The American Cancer Society's *Guidelines for Cancer Related Checkup: Recommendations and Rationale* states, "In 1972, a National Academy of Sciences (BEIR-NAS) report estimated that every rad of radiation delivered to the breast causes approximately six new cases of breast cancer per million women per year after a ten-year delay."[11]

For most other x-rays, our chests are carefully shielded from radiation spill. Yet with mammography we are given a direct dose to each breast along with reassurances that it is safe. Sensitive organs such as the thymus gland (located near the breast bone), the thyroid, and the ovaries for women of childbearing age may require some type of shield. The thymus gland is not considered, even though it is responsible for immunological development and it is a reservoir for cancer-fighting T-cells. I never see radiologists stand in the same room when the mammography machine is operating, yet they assure their clients that very little or no radiation scatter is associated with mammography.

Information control is another way women's decision-making ability is influenced by government policy and funding. Informing women about what questions they should ask before going in for a mammogram would be a public service, since medicine has demonstrated its reluctance about accurately representing the limitations or the risks of today's technology. For example, during the Bush Administration government agencies acquiesced to a gag rule preventing doctors from discussing abortion alternatives in federally funded health centers, continued to balk at requiring oral-contraceptive package inserts that clearly represent the risks, remained quiet about the lack of breast-implant safety information from manufacturers who produce saline implants; they aren't likely to initiate a policy for reporting mammography-safety guidelines to the public.

Women can ask for some information on the phone when scheduling their mammogram:

1. Is the mammography unit a dedicated unit? This means the machine is used for one purpose only, rather than for multiple uses. Dedicated machines provide the highest-quality images.
2. How many mammography units does the center have? You need to know this before you ask about radiation levels, to know whether you will be using the unit with the lowest levels. If there is more than one unit, you will need results for each unit.
3. When was the machine last tested by a physicist? The American College of Radiology (ACR) accreditation program requires that machines be inspected annually. Not all facilities meet ACR standards. Sometimes more time passes than technicians realize. One facility I contacted refused to give me any data because it had been so long since their unit had been tested. Make a note of the date of the most recent report while you're at it. Then when you call next year you will be able to compare the answers, knowing approximately what time of year the machine will be calibrated. You may want to consider scheduling future appointments soon after inspection time.
4. What is the mean-glandular-dose indicated on the physicist's most recent report? This will be a per-view number. It might be quoted as millirads (one thousand millirads equals one rad) or grays. Grays are a new unit of measure, almost equivalent to rads. The facilities I contacted ranged from 60 millirads to 212 millirads per view. This

value multiplied by four views, indicates a 250 percent difference in radiation levels, which makes a substantial difference in the long-term effect. A chest x-ray is ten to twenty millirads per view. Mammograms in the early 1970s were four thousand millirads (four rads) per view. Today's radiation levels are therefore considered low by this standard but relatively high when compared with a chest x-ray.

5. Is the facility accredited? If the answer is yes, you won't need to ask additional questions about image quality and clinical expertise. These standards must be met to receive accreditation. If it is not accredited, you will need to ask more questions:
   a. What was the image-quality score indicated on the physicist's report? Two kinds of phantoms are used. One is provided by the FDA, the other by ACS, and they have different scoring standards. To meet ACR standards, ten is a minimum score but the objects must be uniformly distributed to pass. By FDA standards, eight out of a total of sixteen is considered a satisfactory image. The higher the number the better the quality. The use of a grid increases image quality, but it also requires more radiation. You may want to ask if a grid was used when the phantom was tested. Younger women have denser breast tissue. Denser breasts, or breasts that have had multiple biopsies and have scars, also require more radiation. Density and scar tissue can make images more difficult to read. Screening mammograms are not recommended for asymptomatic women under forty. If a symptom develops, then a diagnostic mammogram or a sonogram might be requested by your doctor.
   b. The American College of Radiology recommends that facilities that are not accredited be asked the following questions regarding training: Is the radiologist who reads the mammogram specially trained to do so? Is the person providing the mammogram a registered technologist? How long has the technologist been working at this facility?

Anticipate some resistance to your requests, because this is not the kind of information mammography centers want to make public. Information about image quality and radiation levels is often not available to the receptionist, so you will need to speak to the chief radiologist or manager. Don't be surprised if you are asked to call back. If a facility refuses outright to give this information, ask your doctor to get it for you or to recommend another facility. Our desire to become informed will help the professionals recommending the use of this technology to also become better informed.

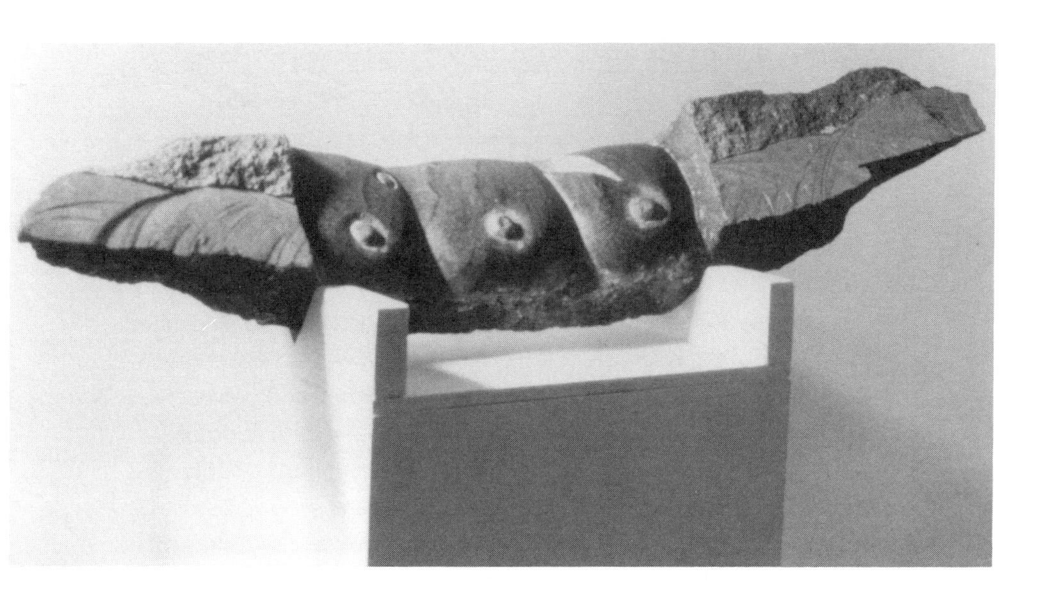

Cancer Fears No. 2
Jill A. Lion, Baltimore, Maryland
Soapstone, 9½" x 46" x 8", 1989

"My maternal grandmother had breast cancer. In my 40s, I had discomfort from a fibrocystic condition in both breasts. I had annual mammograms. At age 47, I had a needle biopsy. . . . In 1991, at 49 years old, I needed a surgical biopsy on each breast. . . . In 1992, at 50 years old, I needed another surgical biopsy (L breast). . . . This time, the diagnosis was lobular carcinoma in situ *with involvement of ducts. My surgeon recommended a double mastectomy. She said I now had a 30 percent chance of developing breast cancer. . . . I miss my breast, but I don't miss the terror of the possibility of having breast cancer."*

Ultimately women need to find facilities that offer the best images, the lowest levels of radiation, and the best technology for providing the most accurate results. Short of legislating quality control, which is in the works, each woman needs to become a responsible consumer of x-rays.

Any screening promotion also runs the risk of increasing incidence due to the "fear factor." Fear of a disease is a powerful influence—as evidenced by many a medical student who develops phantom symptoms. Fear of breast cancer, which caused more women to seek exams, has been attributed to the sharp rise in the incidence in 1974, the year Betty Ford and Happy Rockefeller told the world that they had breast cancer.

The power of the mind cannot be underestimated—an observation that goes hand in hand with recognizing the influence and persuasiveness of advertising. I hate to think for even a minute that exploitation of women's fear of a disease like breast cancer has become a popular marketing strategy, but nonetheless, some politicians support breast-cancer issues in an effort to market themselves to women voters, and some health providers use mammography as a high-profile marketing tool to attract new patients into the medical system.

Mammography as a diagnostic tool is not something toward which women are naturally inclined. Few women willingly want to subject their breasts to radiation and sometimes painful compression. The basic design of this test goes against common sense. Yet women health care providers and volunteers are eagerly telling women patients that it's all right, it doesn't hurt, or if it does it's worth it; the radiation isn't harmful and when you understand the benefits you won't mind a little discomfort.

Where is such rhetoric coming from? In 1991, the United States government began spending more than fifty million of our tax dollars every year because the large cancer-industry-supported organizations and institutions with mammography facilities lobbied to tell women that screening was good for them.[12] All these valuable promotional dollars could be used for research into the causes of breast cancer. They could be used to find a less traumatic treatment that provides better results. Or they could be used to develop better detection technology that doesn't use radiation. But until we can demonstrate that it is financially beneficial to *prevent* breast cancer, we will be stuck with a misrepresented early-detection program. Why, you ask? Doctors and FDA scientists simply keep repeating, "This is the best we have."

In prevention studies, drugs (like tamoxifen for healthy high-risk[13] women) are championed over more benign alternatives that could achieve similar results. The role of tamoxifen is to reduce estrogen production in women. An extremely low-fat diet (less than 15 percent) also lowers estrogen production. This kind of trial is less likely to be supported because there isn't a drug company behind it, pushing to increase the demand for its product by showing positive results. Tamoxifen costs about two dollars per day, and the cost continues to rise as demand and research are increased. "Healthy high-risk women" may need to take this drug for the rest of their lives—it's just like paying a tax for being women. In the meantime, as happened with birth-control pills, healthy women are being used as guinea pigs to test yet another hormone-influencing drug.

Far more profit potential exists in enrolling new patients in treatment programs than in promoting prevention. At some point it would become economically unsound to leave the doctors waiting for new patients and the mammography machines idle. In the *American Journal of Epidemiology*, David Skegg argues that "more frequent surveillance"—annual visits to the doctor—may increase the number of oral-contraceptive users identifying more lumps.[14] Attempting to demonstrate this as a bias in case-control studies, he states, "Breast lumps which although *histologically defined as malignant*, are in fact *biologically benign* [emphasis added] and might never otherwise have come to attention." Other researchers have also suggested that all malignant lumps will not necessarily pose a threat to the patient's life and can inflate survival statistics because conventional diagnosis and treatment were applied to patients who would have survived anyway.[15] It is not unusual for breast tumors to be discovered during an autopsy of patients who died of other causes, unaware that they had a malignant breast mass. Likewise, many lesions diagnosed as a result of biopsies of one breast following a mastectomy for cancer of the other breast would not have shown up clinically as disease during the woman's lifetime. All of these examples point to the more general possibility that "the increasingly vigorous search for lumps, with detection of lesions that are histologically cancerous but biologically benign, [is] an explanation for the occurrence of suddenly large increases in the recorded incidence of breast cancer without concomitant increases in mortality."[16]

ISSUES OF SAFETY ARE POLITICAL

The Food and Drug Administration (FDA) is responsible for ensuring the safety of medical devices and drugs. FDA regulation covers breast implants, quality of mammograms, oral contraceptives, hormone-replacement therapy, BST (bovine growth hormone), tamoxifen, and chemotherapy. The FDA also works in coordination with other government agencies like the Centers for Disease Control (CDC) and the National Cancer Institute (NCI).

When women started to associate distant health problems—arthritis, autoimmune disorders, and migraines—with silicone-filled breast implants, the FDA asked manufacturers for data to demonstrate that these adverse incidents were not associated with the implants. Battle lines formed. These implants have been in use for more than thirty years and are used by two million women.[17] Approximately 20 percent are used for reconstruction in women who have had breast cancer, and the majority are used for augmentation purposes.

First the argument centered on depriving cancer patients of this option to preserve their self-esteem. Then it shifted to a "freedom of choice" platform, assertions being made that women should have the right to choose whether they want to take this risk. Unfortunately, two million women already have made this choice without scientific data to support the implant's safety.

No doctor or patient can be certain of the safety of the implants because the data do not exist. The manufacturers have not conducted satisfactory studies. The studies provided before the hearings did not include large samples of women and followed users for only two years.

Political pressure, including a $4 million campaign mounted by a lobbying group called the American Society of Plastic and Reconstruction Surgeons, Inc., resulted in the FDA panel's initial unanimous recommendation that the implants should remain available, despite inadequate supporting data even after ten years of consideration about implants. This nonbinding recommendation was reversed in April 1992 (after Dr. Kessler, the director of the FDA, declared a moratorium on implants), permitting their use only for study purposes in women who lose a breast as a result of cancer. This compromise position came after a member of Congress, herself a victim of breast cancer, testified that she had already begun the reconstruction process before the moratorium was declared.

She was familiar with the evidence and still believed she should have the option of using silicone implants.

According to the National Cancer Institute, private industry studies are the most difficult to monitor, since these project results are available only when they are "volunteered." For example, many drugs may be tested by a drug company before it discovers one that offers positive results. In the meantime all the other findings—information that might be learned from the "failures"—is kept in private files, as was demonstrated by the investigations of the implant manufacturers!

ISSUES OF FUNDING ARE DEFINITELY POLITICAL

Women of the baby-boom generation are now reaching menopause and the age when they become more at risk for breast cancer. This is a well-educated, consumer-oriented generation that is demanding a greater role in its health-care decisions. As a result these women are forming activist groups and coalitions such as the National Breast Cancer Coalition. They are organizing marches, rallies, and letter-writing campaigns to demand changes in how breast cancer is advertised, diagnosed, and treated while asking for more investment in prevention.

Initially the cry was against the local medical establishment around quality-of-care issues. This early awareness was quickly transferred to the national arena once it became apparent that doctors were limited by the research available to them. My initial reaction was to wonder why my doctor wasn't asking for better techniques. Why wasn't my doctor testifying on behalf of women? Soon I understood that it is unusual and difficult for doctors to be both researchers and clinicians. They are limited by the hours in the day and cannot do both; neither do they have the time to be activists.

Women breast-cancer activists, therefore, are doing their own homework, speaking to Congress and the National Institutes of Health about how research dollars are allocated, in order to ensure that breast cancer is not ignored as it has been in the past. For instance, the National Cancer Institute (NCI) is one of the largest-funded research organizations in the United States. The institute is awarded more than $200 billion a year and uses the services of thousands of volunteers. Yet, although it maintains an enormous information database, there is no particular group at this well-funded, well-staffed organization that acts as a "think tank" to analyze the

VOTE FOR YOURSELF
DEMAND A CURE
DEMAND PREVENTION
1992 MATUSCHKA
BREAST CANCER KILLS WOMEN

WHAM!
Women's Health Action & Mobilization
P.O. Box 733, New York, NY 10009
(212) 713-5966

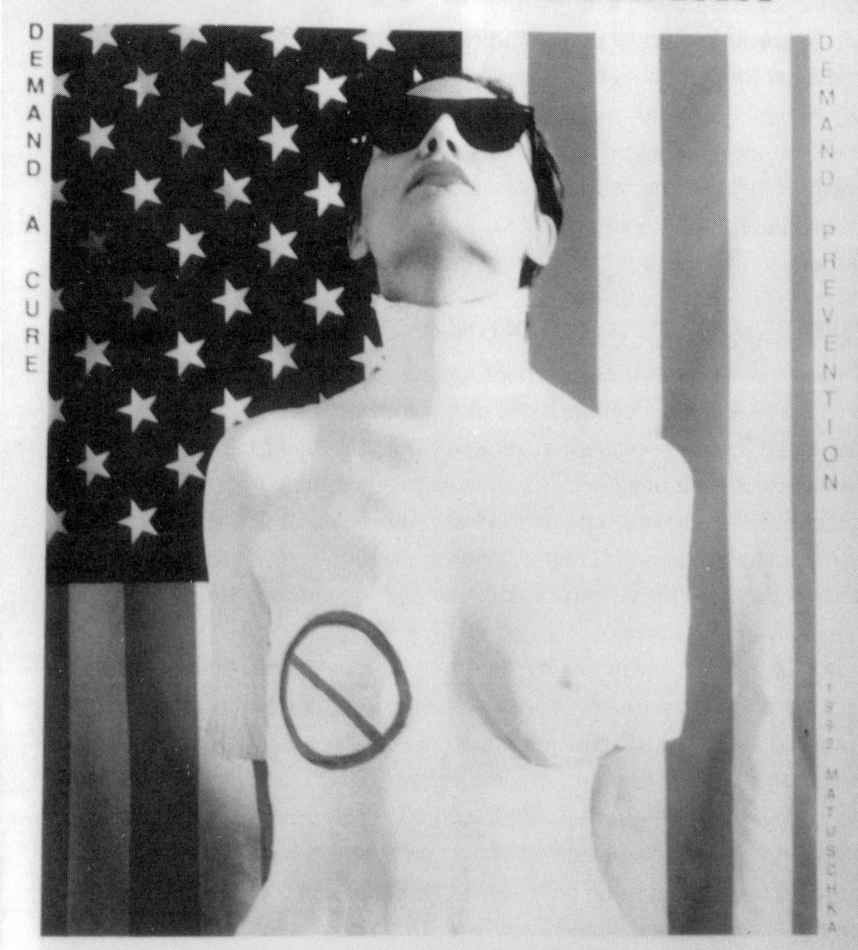

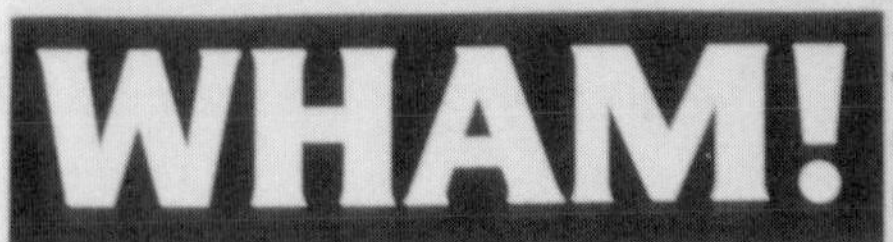

Vote for Yourself
Matuschka, New York, New York
35 mm color "C" print as poster, 16" x 20", 1991

huge volume of new data generated by the NCI in an attempt to assemble some larger picture.

Can you imagine trying to build a space shuttle this way, with fragments of the assembly plan designed and drawn by different scientists all around the country? Imagine the chaos if each part were built and tested but all the parts were never brought together at one site, and no one person or organization knew what the finished space ship would look like or how it would function? Yet, for a disease of the magnitude of breast cancer, we have no center that brings together every research link that now exists. In fact, any scientists who don't conform to the traditional areas of exploration are considered "kooks" and unworthy of serious consideration.

While the FDA oversees drug and medical-device safety, the United States Department of Health compiles statistics reported by the various research organizations and publishes reports like *Cancer Rates and Risks.* Nevertheless, those data are usually not up-to-date; they have a four- to six-year lag time. The research being conducted today focuses on individual frontiers, each scientist hoping that he or she will be able to solve the puzzle by discovering the missing piece. What seems particularly curious about the way research is funded is the process by which grants are supported. Endless questions and possibilities are raised; but the projects most likely to get funding are the ones that advance some aspect of what is already obvious. For example, if a particular drug is determined to be toxic and cause other cancers or heart failure, then researchers look at every combination of varied doses, duration, age of patients it is administered to, combinations with other drugs that will offset toxic or heart-weakening effects, and so on. One drug might be studied for forty years with no significant results, but as long as scientists follow a line of research that has already been developed, they can get research grants for years and years.

To give some historical perspective to funding you should know that for fiscal year 1990, Congress allocated $81 million for all breast-cancer research to the National Cancer Institute; $17.3 million was tagged for basic research into the origin of this disease.[18] By contrast, AIDS research received $2.2 billion[19]—twenty-seven times as much (with $892 million for research). The imbalance was heightened by the fact that during the years 1981 through 1990, about eighty-one thousand people died of

AIDS,[20] while in the same period more than four hundred thousand women died of breast cancer.[21]

According to statistics released in November 1991, "the nation's medical bill for treating people with AIDS or HIV will reach $5.8 billion this year, while the annual cost of treating people with all cancers is estimated to be $35.5 billion. The average per patient cost of treatment for AIDS is $32,000;[22] the cost for Stage I breast cancer averages $25,000 per patient.[23]

If mammograms cost fifty dollars, the revenue generated by medical facilities in screening an estimated thirty-one million women over the age of fifty is about $1.5 billion per year.[24] Looking at these figures leaves little doubt that health care is an industry and that prevention of disease would have an economic impact. Heath care currently makes up more than 12 percent of the gross national product. AIDS activism has helped to radicalize breast-cancer patients by providing a model for getting attention and needed funding. However, breast-cancer patients are quick to point out that we are not competing for the same dollars as AIDS. The focus of debate is not on how the health-care pie is divided but on how to increase the size of the pie—a primary thrust in breast-cancer activism is directed toward gaining new dollars from the defense budget. This new breed of activist is using more feminine metaphors to get their message across, such as "It's time to re-bake this pie."

BREAST CANCER ACTIVISM

The 1.6 million women living with breast cancer are beginning to give this disease a face and a voice, refusing to remain private about it and effecting a change in how breast cancer is treated by organizing in grassroots groups. Not everyone wants to "join" a movement. Some want to act independently. Still others are jockeying for spotlight positions. But all these players have an important contribution to make because of their personal experience. Every woman who has had breast cancer is now an expert. She has had an experience that qualifies her to have an opinion about this subject. Her point of view is as important as her doctor's. How can these women work together?

In 1991 the National Breast Cancer Coalition (NBCC) was founded by six organizations. In only seven months the coalition grew to 137 member organizations. This appears to be the start of a new era in awareness. Dr. Susan Love, in her lectures around the country, is giving women cause and permission to be outrageous and to express their anger. The primary purpose of the coalition is to support research in, access to, and influence over that which will lead to the eradication of breast cancer. For the first time, breast-cancer survivors have a voice at the national table that will influence future research policy.

The unusual mix of organizations represented by the coalition includes the National Alliance of Breast Cancer Organizations, Y-Me National, and the American Cancer Society—all national cancer organizations; grassroots organizations such as the Mary-Helen Mautner Project for Lesbians with Cancer in Washington, D.C., the Virginia Breast Cancer Foundation in Richmond, Virginia, the Women's Community Cancer Project in Cambridge, Massachusetts; and women's groups like the American Jewish Congress and the Fund for the Feminist Majority, along with hospitals and medical institutes.

In the first five months of the organization's history, a national letter writing campaign collected and delivered 600,000 letters to Congress and President Bush. Our original goal had been 175,000 letters, which represented the number of women to be diagnosed that year. Although President Bush did not personally receive or acknowledge the letters, Congress responded with an immediate $40 million increase to the 1992 NCI's breast cancer research budget. The overall increase from $102 million to $142 million was considered a substantial accomplishment in a year when insiders were saying there was no extra money. AIDS activists, however, helped us put into perspective the insignificance of this increase by reminding us that one major study would cost about $250 million. But because it had been so long since *any* increase was made in breast cancer research, female members of Congress felt encouraged that women had made a commitment to come to Washington to fight for this cause.

In January 1992, Congressman Bernard Sanders from Vermont introduced a major piece of cancer research legislation known as the Cancer Registries Act. The bill was inspired by the Breast Cancer Action Group, a visionary grassroots organization in Vermont of which I am the president and co-founder, in order to find out why Vermont's death rates were so high. No one could answer this question because cancer patients are not tracked. Much to everyone's dismay I was able to demonstrate that we know more about the histories of our baseball players than we do about cancer patients. The Cancer Registries Act creates a uniform system of collecting data on all cancer patients so that more epidemiology can occur.

The legislation was passed by the Senate under the care of Senator Leahy, also from Vermont, and passed the House in late spring. Unfortunately it was attached to a larger bill for women's health research that included fetal tissue research, so President Bush vetoed the whole package. This, however, was not the end of the story.

The legislation was reintroduced in October 1992 before the session closed and passed both the House and Senate. Bush signed it into law before the November election, and President Clinton has helped to fund this long overdue program. It's difficult to believe that such basic data gathering and management would need to be grassroots inspired!

In February 1992 another success story began. A special hearing was organized by the NBCC to determine what research wasn't being done and to create a budget for new funding. The conclusion was that $300 million more would open up new opportunities for research. Initially this additional funding had been part of the bill that was vetoed by President Bush.

NBCC's strategy was to get funding from the Department of Defense. We had wanted to take advantage of the fact that it was an election year, however we could not have ordered a more favorable sequence of events. The Berlin Wall and Soviet Union had fallen, the Tailhook scandal was haunting both Congress and the navy, and President Bush wasn't looking very good in the polls. This combination of circumstances permitted Senator Tom Harkin to introduce legislation to direct funds formerly used for national defense, toward civilian purposes. It also was a time when no Congress member wanted to be seen as voting against a women's issue as nonpartisian as breast cancer. The legislation passed through Congress easily, possibly with the unspoken hope that everyone could look good while the president would quietly kill it. This, however, didn't happen.

When the activists got wind that the Office of Budget and Management was going to remove this item from the defense budget and place it into the domestic budget, in effect killing it when the domestic budget wouldn't balance, phone calls, telegrams, and letters poured in. What was supposed to be a secret way of killing legislation that didn't appear to harm anyone's chances of getting reelected was now becoming a presidential problem. They could not take this action with the public watching right before what was now forecast to be a close election.

At the eleventh hour, much to everyone's astonishment, including the Department of Defense, $210 million of "earmarked" funds for breast cancer research was passed *within* the Department of Defense's budget. We all learned a lot about how our government works and how programs get funded through this experience. It was also during this fight that we realized it was not enough to send new funds into the system. We saw a real need to have patient advocates play an active role in overseeing how the funds were spent.

With this in mind, our 1993 efforts focused on getting a "comprehensive strategy to end the epidemic." This time 2.6 million signatures were collected and presented to President Clinton. As a result of the nationwide effort, the president instructed the Department of Health and Human Services to hold a "summit "on how to end the breast cancer epidemic. Experts and activists were invited to share their vision about what needed to be done. Recommendations were gathered into a report; however, after a few drafts, important language and suggestions disappeared. As has been typical with our government agencies, revised reports are sent out for comment right before a holiday weekend, which limits our ability to respond with the necessary impact. The NBCC activists are now negotiating to recover the fruits of their work.

As Dr. Samuel Broder, director of the National Cancer Institute, once remarked, "It takes time to turn around an aircraft carrier." The people in government are satisfied to move along at the pace they have for decades, and although the work of activists has demonstrated that we can garner increased attention and funding, it still remains to be seen if having these dollars is the answer to ending the epidemic.

Alisa Solomon observes that cancer is a disease with a much longer history than, for example, AIDS:

> a history that includes huge institutions, a deeply entrenched bureaucracy, expenditures of tens of billions of dollars, a longstanding public campaign promoting specific conceptions and responses to the disease, and millions of deaths. New cancer activism, unlike AIDS

activism, must position itself in relation to a wide range of already functioning organizations and already ingrained public perceptions.[25]

Dr. Samuel Epstein, author of *The Politics of Cancer,* thinks that under the present system, women's groups are in fact being "conned into demanding more funds for the NCI." He points out that "executives from agribusiness, pharmaceutical, petrochemical, and even tobacco companies often sit on the boards of major cancer-research institutions." Their presence encourages scientists toward developing "treatments that will be profitable for drug manufacturers, while they shy away from finding preventions."[26] In the words of Judith Brady, author of *1 in 3 Women with Cancer Confront an Epidemic,* pushing for more money for the NCI without pushing for a whole new direction is "throwing good money after bad. They're barking up the wrong tree."[27]

These words aren't limited to the most radical thinkers, either. John Bailar, M.D., professor of epidemiology and biostatistics at McGill University in Montreal, and formerly with the National Cancer Institute, states, "Perhaps the biggest misstep so far has been the failure to emphsize cancer prevention. The government spends only one dollar on cancer-prevention research for every three dollars it spends on cancer-treatment research. It's time to reverse that spending ratio."[28]

No idea is more threatening to the intertwined interests of government bureaucracy and business than a visible display by women activists such as the one put forth by Audre Lorde, of "an army of one-breasted women descending on Congress and demanding that the use of carcinogenic, fat-stored hormones in beef-feed be outlawed."[29] Although I have met few women who would be comfortable with this kind of public display, the possibility alone has provided the necessary incentive for giving attention to this cause. More women's groups are becoming involved in learning about breast cancer. Finally, women have become willing to demonstrate their growing impatience. They aren't waiting another generation for scientists to tell them what to do. What role you and I play in the reform of women's health-care delivery depends on our health, guts, support, and vision of a different reality.

To assure that we have the health to fight this fight we need to take control of what we put in our bodies that could prove to be detrimental to us. This includes the kind of food and water we consume, the types of drugs and figure-altering devices we use, and even the messages we hear and internalize about how we will feel in the near future. If women are told that by year 2000 one in six women will have breast cancer, this will likely come true. If we demand that politicians and the medical organizations who want to exploit breast cancer accurately represent the present reality, rather than forecasting the future, then we become proactive in stopping self-fulfilling prophecies. We can choose to advocate for an honest reality, walk around flat-chested with dignity, say what we feel about the tragedy of breast cancer as it exists now, and garner respect for our convictions. We can choose to use what remaining life we have for promoting women's issues.

For a while I considered going back to graduate school to become an epidemiologist. I wanted to conduct my own research, since no one else seemed to be doing the kind of studies we need to prevent breast cancer. I wanted to study the effects of dairy consumption on world populations and cluster populations. I wanted to look at the effects of radiation on long-term survival and the effects of oral contraceptives on risk of breast cancer. But then I learned that getting an advanced degree would only tie me to a system with standards and rules that haven't helped other scientists with similar dreams. Having a Ph.D. or an M.D. doesn't always open doors, and in fact can close doors, because in order to achieve professional ranking many women are being trained to conform to and to advocate the party line. In essence they are silenced by the very system they wanted to help advance.

By staying outside this system, I am freer to think and say what I wish. Speaking from my heart on a subject that I feel so deeply about is the hardest part of this work. It would have been so much easier to just go to the surgeon and have the cancer cut out, and then go about my old, comfortable life, ignoring the issues, denying the hurt. But I feel a responsibility to be vocal.

Today when I talk about breast cancer I often find myself screaming, speaking loudly, forcefully, angrily; I sense I'm not being heard. It's as though there isn't enough space or time for me to say all that needs to be said. The urgency I feel is brought on by sharing the dying experience of my new cancer friends. We were all fine, fighting the disease, fighting for the cause, riding our bikes together, having potluck dinners, sharing stories. Then one by one we die. I often wonder whether I can do this.

Can I continue in my work as an activist, as a writer, and watch my friends fall? I feel so helpless; these deaths are so senseless. Five women die every hour of every day from breast cancer in this country, and it seems as though no one notices.

So many people I speak to look at me blankly and say, "But all cancer is a tragedy. Why do you think breast cancer is special?" As long as it is not a national priority, the breast cancer epidemic will remain a metaphor for how society treats women. I want to see and hear more women enraged by this indignity.

Is fighting the disease on a social and political level good for our health? I find the answers to this question in the women who live in my community, the people who call me because their friend, mother, or sister was just diagnosed. They want more information, and they aren't satisfied with what the doctor has to say. Presently there aren't enough people to turn to who will provide information on how to make our own health-restoring choices.

As my research files grow with information about the many causes associated with breast cancer, I become increasingly discouraged, knowing that I live in a country that is perpetuating more disease than it can counteract, let alone heal. I have a difficult time understanding how we as a nation can have so many government regulatory bodies and still be so naive about the risks imposed by electromagnetic and ionizing radiation as well as by carcinogens.

In 1990 I wrote an article published in the *Burlington Free Press* calling for a closer look at the causes of breast cancer. The local medical community went crazy. For more than a month after publication, numerous letters from doctors and their supporters appeared in the paper discrediting me and my facts. Essentially the outcry said, "Don't take away the hope that women can be cured." Doctors defended their myth, stating that great strides have been made in treating this disease.

At the same time, however, other physicians like Susan Love began coming forward to say that the emperor has no clothes: We still don't know how to prevent or treat breast cancer. Although the people who work in the cancer industry think women should be more grateful for the changes that have occurred—they always emphasize, "It could be worse"—activists are asking, "Why isn't it much better after all this time?" Breast cancer was the first cancer to be discovered—in the fifth century

B.C.E.—and unlike polio, scurvy, or tuberculosis, breast-cancer incidence has never shown a significant decrease. Over the years the list of risk factors has grown, but we are still in the dark about how this disease can be prevented.

Each woman must do something to change this situation. As women, we must find the power to not feel shame about who we are. The shame women feel may well be a by-product of our continued collective denial about how brutal breast-cancer treatment remains, an apparent legacy of Saint Agatha's torture. But we can stop the abandonment. We can stop the dependency. In the 1960s women reportedly burned their bras and demanded their freedom. Now almost thirty years later we must fight with similar intensity to save our breasts and our lives.

My dream for the future is for our outcry to start to influence political elections. Politicians and presidents must realize that if they do not make the elimination of breast cancer a national priority they will not be reelected to office.

People are the nervous system of politicians, and government funding is the blood supply to national prevention programs. Women uniting together around this cause can become the heart of our nation's new health-care system. As women awaken to this new role as expectant health-conscious consumers, the whole nation will reap the benefits. On a global level, allowing breast cancer to ravage women is equivalent to destroying all the mountains on earth.

My dream is for all the environmental and hormonal causes of breast cancer to be identified and made public by the end of the 1990s and for an aggressive prevention program to be funded and instituted. My dream is for all the women who are diagnosed with breast cancer to have psychological and physical rehabilitation programs as a standard part of their covered patient care. My dream is for screening and treatment programs that don't involve compression, radiation, or other abusive and potentially cancer-producing techniques.

My dream is for a cleaner environment and a sensitivity to the bidirectional relationship between health and disease—to the realization that disease is a warning to us to pay closer attention to our planet. Health-care professionals can no longer just treat symptoms. This approach is bankrupting our system. We need to become more capable of seeing relationships and understanding illness mechanisms. Some doctors have treated women as the ignorant gender, but I look forward to a time when the male model on which these ideas have been based will crumble. If enough women abandon the system to seek their own health-restorative path, the system will change.

Women have good instincts. Now we must learn how to trust them and not be so easily convinced that the doctor knows best. I have explained how I approached this problem so that others can see that there are options, but not necessarily so that other women will follow my path. My path was not direct; I had to discover for myself what the options were. I hope other women can use what I have learned as background to go even further and to uncover more options.

Womankind is under threat of extinction. At the current rate of increase in incidence, by the year 2010 every woman alive will expect to have breast cancer at some time during her life. Women at risk are being given drugs such as tamoxifen that induce menopause-like symptoms; they are being encouraged to have their ovaries removed; they are offered prophylactic breast removal. How far away from "medically necessary sterilization" are we for a unilateral solution to both breast cancer and the abortion question? Scientists are already trying to develop drugs to genetically inoculate women against breast cancer. Yet, the long-term effects of genetic engineering may not be fully understood for another thirty years.

In an attempt to halt the rampage of certain hormones in women's bodies, our reproductive systems are being attacked on several fronts—with genetics, with surgery, with other hormones, and in politics. Meanwhile, science is moving further and further from the simple truth.

As a society we must take responsibility for sowing the seeds of epidemic breast cancer. To stop cultivating this epidemic we have to pay attention to the planet and every single life form on it, starting right now.

Epilogue

It's been two years since I completed the text of this book, and five years since my diagnosis. During this time I have achieved many personal goals: the development of a small, state-wide, nonprofit organization, the Breast Cancer Action Group, into a nationally recognized organization; the initiation and passage of the Cancer Registry Act of 1992, which will create a uniform system of collecting information on cancer patients throughout the United States; the passage of earmarked "parallel" funding for breast cancer research in the Department of Defense; the organization of the first conference to speak to women with breast cancer about the psychosocial issues of breast cancer; the creation of the first tribute to women who have died from breast cancer, "The Face of Breast Cancer: A Photographic Essay"; and the creation of an arts registry for women with breast cancer, "Healing Legacies: A Collection of Art and Writing by Women with Breast Cancer," which premiered at the U.S. House of Representatives in October 1993. I have also learned that true healing goes beyond the political.

For me this journey has not been a straight or calculated path. I have wandered for some time through the forest of journals, libraries, doctors' offices, diagnostic tests, research institutions, political obstacles, and cancer recurrences and losses. As I emerge on the other side of this morass I feel quite certain that the way breast cancer is diagnosed and treated is archaic and harmful to both patients and caregivers. This fear-based, disempowering system needs a complete overhaul. I believe this overhaul needs to be directed by vision, not science. For until we have a vision of what we need, it cannot be so. All that I have accomplished has begun with a clear vision of the result I wanted.

My vision for the future is that women will be empowered to become sensitive to their own bodies and take responsibility for their own healing. Our survival and success is contingent on our willingness to turn inward for our healing. The tests used to diagnosis breast cancer are horribly inadequate. Mammograms still only diagnosis 30 to 40 percent of breast cancer cases. Blood tests, CAT scans, and bone scans—used as follow-up measures after a woman's diagnosis—do not detect recurrence at its earliest stages. Chemotherapy is a mystery. No one really knows how or why it works, whom it will benefit, and for how long. Radiation is a local treatment, and like chemotherapy has significant long- and short-term side effects. Surgery, still the quickest way to rid our bodies of these mutated, fast-multiplying cells, is both crude and assaultive. Scientists and doctors continue to go over and over this same territory as if they had missed some morsel of information that will unlock this complex puzzle. The design of research studies forces scientists to follow the same paths regardless of results. Scientific standards, although strict, do not inspire or support genuine breakthroughs, which in fact seem to happen more by accident than by design.

No one person or institution is to blame for this rut we are currently in. Advances are limited only by our collective vision. Unfortunately, our vision is limited by our fear: fear of death, fear of not getting a research grant, fear of being professionally ostracized for not following standard practice. It seems to be of no concern that these standards are based on faulty basic premises. It is time—no, it is past time—for us to stop yielding our consciousness to the costly cancer research and treatment industry that has not been able to provide a significant method for reducing the increase in new cases or mortality in the past sixty years.

When I turn inward for answers I am told that my breast cancer is not an issue of life or death. My breast cancer is about discovering how to take better care of my body while creating physical and spiritual environments for personal healing and transformation to occur. During my own journey I learned about the importance of diet, yoga, and release of emotional insults that I carry around in my cells. I discovered life beyond my present understanding. I explored my past lives to reveal my true life's purpose. I talked to spiritual guides and challenged their advice. I learned to trust my inner voice, to sharpen my hearing to what it tells me, and to believe that this is not a trick of my imagination.

Breast cancer, like other cancers, holds for us spiritual messages. A few messages have been repeated to me many times. The underlying message is that healing breast cancer is essentially about transformation: transformation of both cells and soul. Like water, which can be solid when frozen, crystalline as snow, and fluid when melted, our cells can take on other forms and can also return to their previous composition. Cells are influenced by more than heat and cold; they are also influenced by invisible energies and environmental stimulants.

We can of course cut them out, burn them, poison them, and think we are done with it—or we can get in touch with why we have cancer and transform it into an incredibly valuable learning about ourselves and creation. Cells are composed of energy. Attacking cancer is a form of dishonoring and disowning our bodies. Pumping chemicals and radiation into our cells distances us even further from feeling our life force.

Transformation instead needs to occur on three energetic levels: physical, emotional, and spiritual. True healing requires an investment of energy on all three levels. Our medical system is simply not set up to treat people in a holistic way. It is up to us as individuals to take responsibility for using medicine as just one of many techniques for treating our physical self, and to spend equal time and energy on other approaches such as cleaning up our diet and our living and working environments; using bodywork and emotional catharsis to release old anger, fear, and pain that are stored in our cells; and listening attentively to our inner voice, which holds many gifts of wisdom.

Another message I have heard over and over again is that what we believe and think influences our healing. Individually we are all creators. We have the ability to create our own reality. This can occur on either a conscious or an unconscious level. If we choose to be in touch with our inner voice, than we can make conscious choices about our health and our life in general. Psychic healing and psychic surgery are not just New Age terms. This type of healing has occurred throughout history. Our belief system is our only limitation to utilizing this gift.

Finally, I have learned that the solution to solving the breast cancer puzzle is within us. We, the women who have breast cancer, are the ones with the answers and the knowing. They are not outside. We do not have to wait for solutions to be discovered and sanctioned by someone else. With this deep belief, I propose that regeneration is possible—regeneration of our physical bodies. Science has documented that when arteries to the heart become blocked, our body compensates by creating new pathways for our blood to flow. Norman Cousins talks about this in his book *The Healing Heart.* Deepak Chopra tells the story of a client who refused to have his leg amputated after being electrocuted. This man, in having an out-of-body experience, learned the technique of restoring his life and used this technique to rebuild the nerves and blood vessels in his leg. Two women I know have been able to remove advanced-stage metastasized breast cancer from their bones; they continue to survive today even though their doctors predicted that death was imminent. One woman regenerated two disks in her back. I believe I regenerated my lymph node system, which was severed surgically, causing me to experience lymphedema for one and a half years.

These examples demonstrate to me that regeneration has not only taken place throughout history but takes place today. People are regenerating blood vessels, nerves, bone, and lymph through psychic and spiritual experiences. If this is so, then it is plausible to me that we can consciously decide to regenerate our cells—perhaps even our breasts.

I am compelled to hold out this vision, because when I learned that there is no medical cure for breast cancer, the knowledge undermined my own recovery and, I believe, played a role in my recurrences. For the sake of my continued recovery it has been necessary for me to find another way to frame what I know to be scientifically true. Since I don't feel that ignorance can be a satisfactory option, and since knowledge and education dissolved my dream of a cure, I see the possibility of regeneration as a new avenue of hope.

With this in mind, I invite all women who feel mutilated or less than whole as a result of their breast cancer treatment to move beyond breast cancer and help me demonstrate a new reality. It is you—who like me are so rational that you require a scientific explanation for how you can survive your breast cancer—who like me are seeking a way to be transformed. Together we can hold the possibility of regeneration, using all the means available to us; we can carry with us the responsibility to share our experience with others who are more skeptical so that they too can see a different reality.

We all have the power to see the possibilities in our challenges; to voice our frustration about what is not, and to take steps to create something new—something beyond the average or the expected. The work that lies ahead is to open ourselves to the inner voice and to trust what we hear.

January 1994

Listen

Sometimes I long to shout—
"Stop! Stop the slaughter of our Mother
and of the good and bountiful beauty upon Her!"

this longing, this voice—
within was given to me
by the Great Spirit.
It is the voice of love.

Be silent.
Listen.
From the silence within yourself
you will hear it too.

It is a roar. It is a whisper.
And it is ever present—
waiting to guide you,
if only you will listen.

The voice will reveal to you
to respect your little brothers,
the beauty creatures,
and to preserve the plant and water nations.

From it, you will learn
the friendliness of trees
and not to curse the rain.

Walk in the rain
and be thankful for its goodness.

Give thanks, when our Mother turns her colours—
season to season;

they are beautiful each in their own way
and we also turn and change spinning our part in the cycle.

You will learn that you do not need so many things
and gadgets that you are killing yourselves and your
Mother to obtain.

Everything you need has been provided.
It is here—the voice will tell you—
if only you will listen—

Wi ni napa

Source: Sun Bear, Wabun, Nimimosha and The Tribe, *The Bear Tribe's Self Reliance Book* (Spokane, Wash.: Bear Tribe Publishing Co., 1977).

APPENDIX I

How to Start a Grassroots Organization

There are many reasons for starting your own group. The reason I hear most often is need: you may feel there isn't a group that serves your particular needs, such as support, action, progress, or an exchange of new ideas. If there is more than one person with the same need and you are willing to use your spare time to fill this void, then you have the foundation for a grassroots organization.

The first challenge is to find other women who share the same need or support your desire to have a group. Friends and business associates might be included, and the group need not be limited to people who share your experience with breast cancer. In fact, a mixed group, including women who have not had breast cancer but who feel equally committed to eradicating breast cancer can be very successful.

I found supporters for my thinking and cause by writing an op-ed article for the local newspaper. Op-ed articles appear opposite the newspaper editorial page and frequently reflect the opinions of citizens. Another way to bring people together would be to schedule a meeting with a few friends who have a similar interest and contact the local newspaper to announce that a new group is forming. If a large urban paper does not include these kinds of stories, then use the local throw paper or a community paper.

Talking to oncology nurses and doctors is another way to get in touch with other women like yourself. Women who are in treatment as well as women who come to the office for follow-up can be given a flier or told about your new group. Some doctors are hesitant to promote groups that have a political focus or that do not have a professional facilitator. Most medical professionals are service oriented, and initially they might not see political action as being a service. I wanted to be very clear that my organization was not a support group. My community already has four or five support groups; what we didn't have was a way for women to become active in finding ways to prevent breast cancer from happening to their daughters, sisters, and friends.

In fact, my goal in writing this book is to show how essential social and political issues are in addressing the healing and prevention of this disease. Write down *your* goals. What do you want your group to do that is different from existing groups? What is your ultimate goal? Think big. It's all right to say your goal is to work to eliminate the causes of breast cancer. The large national organizations strive to educate women about "finding cancer," and they work to reduce mortality—save lives—by diagnosing the cancer early. This goal has resulted in the national push for screening mammography. Such programs have raised public awareness about the importance of screening but do nothing to prevent women from getting breast cancer. This is the void I believe needs to be filled. If fewer women get breast cancer, fewer women will die. This is not only a more economical way of reducing mortality, it is also empowering for women. Prevention promotes health. Screening looks for disease. This simple twist in approach resulted in the birth of the breast-cancer grassroots movement.

BUILDING A SUPPORT BASE

What makes grassroots groups different from other organizations is that we represent the patient's perspective. By definition, *grassroots* is "common people, thought of as representing the basic, fundamental source or support" or "society at the local level." Being a community-based organization means that the more supporters you have, the broader your influence. Membership shows your legislators that you represent a particular number of voters. The broader your base, the more influence your group will have with legislators. Community membership may mean a signature on a petition or a one-dollar contribution that says "I want to know how to prevent breast cancer." Ten thousand letters that each have the name and address of a voter who has sent one dollar to your community-based grassroots organization will give your group both a financial base and a constituent base.

Always think in large numbers. Everyone can afford a dollar, and the simpler the message the clearer it will be to the legislators. Fifty-two percent of the American population is female. If every woman sent only one dollar with the message "I want to know how to prevent breast cancer," we would have every representative in the House and Senate working to introduce legislation that would contribute to finding an answer. This is the impact of grassroots. Start your one-dollar campaign by having each person in your group contact ten of her closest friends. Tell these friends either by letter or in person about your group and its mission. Next, ask for a contribution to begin your one-dollar campaign. This seed money will help with postage. Members can ask local businesses to support the cause by donating printing or copying services. I have found more success with firms that have these facilities but are not actually in the printing or copying business. For example, one business in town publishes real-estate directories and has a printer on staff. We provided the paper and camera-ready copy, and they donated the printing service for our first direct-mail piece.

For many people, asking for money is the most difficult element of political organizing. The reality is that people who contribute do so because the issue is important to them. You are not begging; rather, you are providing them with an opportunity to participate in the fight to stop breast cancer.

Monthly meetings allow an organization to be accessible to new members who want to volunteer their time and expertise or just want to learn more about what they can do. I have found that it's best if one person doesn't have to be responsible for sending out meeting notices and holding these meetings. Inviting members to host the meeting in rotation helps everyone to get to know one another better. Notify newspapers that have a section to list meetings. These newspaper listings remind people that the organization is around and growing. We have had better results from personally inviting friends to come to our meetings, and every other month I will add to the meeting announcement, "Bring a friend."

Sometimes minutes are included with the meeting announcement. Always try to include an agenda so people will know what the meeting is about, and try to limit the items on the agenda to an hour and a half to two hours.

In order to raise money you need to incorporate in your state as a nonprofit organization. Each state has a different procedure. Contact the secretary of state in your state capital to find out what you need to do. Some states require only a filing fee and articles of incorporation. The organization president and secretary will be responsible for signing all the forms. Articles of incorporation tell the state the purpose of your organization. Our articles read as follows:

- To promote research into the causes of, cure for, and optimal treatments for breast cancer, through increasing research funding.
- To improve access to high-quality breast-cancer screening, diagnosis, treatment, and care for all women, through legislation and beneficial changes in the regulation and delivery of breast health care.
- To increase the involvement and influence of women living with breast cancer.
- To educate the public about the need to make breast-cancer prevention a national priority.

Feel free to use these for your own articles if you'd like.

The Internal Revenue Service publishes a booklet, *Tax-Exempt Status for Your Organization, Publication 557*. Sections pertaining to 510 (c) (3) status and articles of organization explain how to file for tax-exempt status. This will allow contributors to deduct their donations. A nonprofit organization is considered tax-exempt if the annual gross receipts do not equal more than five thousand dollars. Most organizations can raise money during their first year by only filing for state incorporation—that is, as long as you do not want to apply for grants or raise more than five thousand dollars.

Prepare a written copy of your organization goals and annual objectives. Organization goals are the long-range, ultimate goals of your group. Once your group is up and running—so that you don't end up running in circles, or running out of energy—you will want to focus your objectives. Annual objectives identify what you want to accomplish for the year. For the first year, our annual goals included establishing our organization as a legal entity and doing a direct-mail fund-raiser to help pay our expenses. Filing legal documents costs money even when you are able to get someone to donate legal time to prepare these documents. Other organization goals for our first year were to begin to network with other breast-cancer grassroots organizations nationally and to become known to our federal legislators. We were able to meet our first year goals and exceed our expectations. In October we met to outline our goals for the second year.

Having goals gives an organization focus and direction. When new opportunities come along you can look at your goals and decide: Does this opportunity meet what we want to accomplish? It is impossible to be all things to all people. Knowing what you are helps other people understand better when to call on you.

Some grassroots groups have study groups to learn more about issues. Members identify their questions and then set up groups to research and discuss the literature on those subjects. For example, should a woman with a 0.5-centimeter noninvasive tumor have radiation after lumpectomy? The members divide up the task of researching this question, then meet to discuss their findings. This exercise might produce a policy for your organization about when radiation is and isn't appropriate.

Other grassroots activities might include holding awareness rallies, being available to community speakers bureaus, starting a news-clipping service, producing press releases and press conferences, organizing letter-writing and photo campaigns (the letter writers are encouraged to include a photograph with their letter so the reader has more sense of personal contact), sponsoring races and family days, or setting up awareness and healing conferences. You might eventually become interested in producing a group newsletter or informational pamphlets. Newsletters can be distributed quarterly at first, then six times per year. Pamphlets can be used for promotional mailers and speaker handouts.

Legal and financial advisors are important to consider including in your grassroots organization; it's especially good to have someone with fundraising experience as well as someone with accounting experience. Consider medical advisors, including nurses, epidemiologists, psychotherapists, and doctors. It's also helpful to have political advisors, people who are connected to the leaders in your state.

If your state membership grows quickly, you might want to consider forming chapters so that each region has its own meeting group. You can make your impact felt nationally, too. If possible, ally your organization with national groups like the National Breast Cancer Coalition, the National Women's Health Network, the National Organization for Women, the Older Women's League, and the Women's Political Caucus. Look for organizations that focus on women's issues and that will consider your organization's agenda. Help them see the need to make breast-cancer prevention a priority. When your members go out to speak to these groups, have only two or three key points to discuss about why prevention needs to be a priority. Develop a sales talk and if it works, use it over and over again until your group is recognized as an integral voice in the community.

Develop a list of your United States senators and representatives. Contact each member to let him or her know about your organization and agenda. If you can travel to Washington, this will give you an opportunity to establish rapport with legislative staff members who oversee health issues. The first few trips you may only be scheduled to see the staff members. This is how Washington works. The staff are your representative's eyes and ears—they keep the representative informed of the issues. Don't feel this is second-rate. The support of staff members is equal in importance to the legislator's support. The more often you appear at their door, the more influence you will have.

On your second visit have a particular request in mind. Ask your representative's office for help researching the possibility of some legislation, or discuss some pending legislation. Don't expect them to know the statistics about your cause; they hear about hundreds of good causes. You need to do something to make your cause stand out in their minds. On my first visit, I asked my senators what they were doing to help women in our state. I also asked them if they would be willing to do more. I told them five women were dying every hour in the United States from breast cancer and that no one even knows what is causing these deaths. I reminded them that if there were a mass murderer on the loose killing five women every hour, more would be done, and said that breast cancer needs to be treated like a mass murderer.

Follow up your visits with thank-you notes and information to back up what you discussed. Always think of your request from their perspective. As politicians they want votes, and they need women's votes. Now, what if you decided to let the press know that your representatives had voted against a bill to increase funding for breast-cancer research? Use the press when you want to make your point, but never threaten the legislators. They already have enough fear to contend with, and creating more doesn't necessarily facilitate a working relationship. At the end of each year put together a list of your accomplishments to mail out to your members and legislators.

Above all, have fun with your organization. Gather together people who share similar values and want similar results. Recognize that each person has a special gift to bring to the group, and enjoy everyone's enthusiasm and creativity. If any one person tries to control the group, you can bet that will kill the enthusiasm. Enjoy your involvement and be happy, because life is too short to waste!

GRASSROOTS ORGANIZATION CHECKLIST

- Invite a group of women to an organizational meeting at your home.
- Discuss your interests and see what other women are interested in; decide whether you want to form a formal organization.
- Select a name and designate officers; investigate filing for nonprofit status with the secretary of state.
- Outline your objectives for the first year; do not forget to include fundraising.
- Invite friends of friends to come to future meetings.
- Notify the newspaper about your group. Consider the headline "Pushing for Prevention" for your first news release.
- Do something newsworthy. Organize a rally, speak to local philanthropic organizations, hold a demonstration because you disagree with how your legislators voted on breast-cancer research funding.
- Do something to demonstrate the strength of your organization to your legislators—start a letter-writing campaign or circulate a petition.
- Organize regular monthly meetings, study groups, legislative groups.
- Begin your own news-clipping service. When you disagree with the content of articles or news broadcasts, write about your concerns.
- Implement a fundraising event within the first year.
- File for 501 (c) (3) tax-exempt status and postal nonprofit status six months to a year before you will need it. The government filing takes more time than you might expect.

- Request copies of the following reference publications:

  The Congressional Directory, from the U.S. Government Printing Office, 202-783-3238. There is a charge for this book.

  Cancer Statistics Review, from the National Cancer Institute, 301-496-8510 or 1-800-422-6237. This publication should be complimentary if they know you are a nonprofit organization.

  Cancer Facts & Figures, from the American Cancer Society, 1-800-227-2345. Free.

  Vital & Health Statistics: Breast Cancer Risk Factors and Screening. U.S., 1987, from the National Center for Health Statistics, 301-436-7100.

- Enjoy what you're doing, the people, the cause, and the activities!

APPENDIX 2

A Message for Friends and Families of Women with Breast Cancer

Hearing that I had breast cancer brought on many emotions: fear, grief, anger, deep sadness, hurt, pain, confusion. The reality of this diagnosis is hard to comprehend unless you are actually faced with it. The difficulty in having such a wide range of intense emotions is the loneliness that surrounds them. It feels as though no one else can understand. I wanted to enroll the support of my family and friends; I thought this would give me more confidence in exercising my "right" to decide. I wanted to be surrounded by people who would support me in taking on this huge responsibility. But when I tried to turn to other people for support, their natural responses and my needs didn't particularly match. So if a woman you love is diagnosed with breast cancer, how can you help?

AT THE TIME OF DIAGNOSIS

The natural tendency of family and friends is to ask questions. Although you are well intentioned, by asking questions you trigger other fears with which the newly diagnosed woman may not be ready to cope. In my situation, my sister wanted to know at what stage my cancer was. At that point, I didn't even know breast cancers were staged, and therefore I felt "ignorant" on top of scared. I had just heard I had breast cancer. I wanted love and sympathy. I wanted to know I had support. Who would be there for me? I wasn't asking my friends and relatives for advice yet. I was in need of being held and loved—that's all. No one realized I had this need. So it was a need that remained unmet as I plunged into the nitty-gritty exercise of asking and answering questions pertaining to a disease I knew nothing about.

Now, after years of private therapy, I see I needed time to grieve over what was happening. I needed acknowledgment and caring. I also realize how few people are able to just be present with a grieving individual. It is much more the American way to try to "fix" things—including people and their feelings. Feelings are "made better," not by allowing their expression, but instead by finding ways to distract the attention of the person with the feelings.

I was so sad and so upset that I should have been hysterical and crying, but I wasn't able to have these feelings. No one around me could handle them, and I feared I couldn't handle them alone. The result was that my emotions became knotted up in my throat and chest as I attempted to fit into the role the people around me expected. I helped them with their fears by being strong, but I couldn't help myself. What I needed was to be sad and scared. I just needed to have time to cry.

I also found that when people heard I had cancer they began to treat me as "different" than I was the week before. I was now sick—maybe even dying. The pity was written on their faces. They wanted to help me with things that had nothing to do with my ability or my disease: "Sit down . . . have a danish . . . put your feet up . . . don't move . . . I'll get it for you." It felt as though I had to just quietly accept whatever it was people wanted to offer, whether or not it was appropriate. I had breast cancer, not a broken leg; yet, help often came in this out-of-context form.

I recommend that you try to be present for the woman you love. Be silent yet available, and let her express her fears and needs. Even if she doesn't act as though having breast cancer is any big deal, recognize that this is her way to express feelings based on how they might have been received in her past. Until just recently, I didn't have the kind of person in my life who could allow my feelings to be expressed. I know now why I managed my breast cancer as though it were a business instead of like a deep wound. I was a hurt child in need of comforting, and this was the hardest need to fill because I had few experiences of being comforted.

The night before my mastectomy I was hysterical. I was scared. I didn't know what it would be like; I didn't know if I would ever feel like myself again. When I started crying I was on the floor beside my suitcase. My sister entered the room and told me to get hold of myself, to get up and get ready for bed. I said I needed to be held. "Just get off the floor, and I'll hold you," she said. This was a classic example of our relationship: if I wanted her love I had to have it on her terms. It's taken a lot of interpersonal work to resolve these old feelings and to find the kind of people that could provide the support I needed.

Ultimately the treatment is secondary to coming in touch with our feelings and our friends. There is a special opportunity here for family and friends to relate in a way that they may not have before the diagnosis. Be gentle with the woman who is newly diagnosed, because all the wind has just been knocked out of her. It may be a challenge to accept her pace for asking questions and making decisions during these first few months. This doesn't mean you have to compromise yourself forever. But find a way to process your own fears somewhere else—with an expert or another friend—while she is in this fragile place. Remember, now it's *her* turn to be cared for by *you*.

During the first three months, you can help your friend adjust by being open and loving and by lending a shoulder to cry on. You probably feel that you don't want this person to be hurt or possibly die from breast cancer, and that is something you can openly express; you can be vulnerable too by crying with her. It is important to be clear about your own grief.

If you are crying because of the new obligations put on you it's probably best done elsewhere. Human beings know, on some level, the unconscious level, how the people around them feel. My experience unfortunately included a lot of barriers, distancing, and abandonment. All the time the people around me were saying "I love you. I care," but I didn't feel that inside. I felt from them, "I'm scared. I don't want this to happen to me. What if I get cancer too? What if I'm left taking care of you."

FACING A RECURRENCE

Depending on a person's approach to treatment, a recurrence may or may not be a shock. Many women go through treatment with the impression that once they are treated, that's all there is to it and they'll be fine. It might seem that nothing could be as awful as the shock of receiving the initial diagnosis and then enduring the treatments—that is, until a woman hears that despite all she has been through, the cancer is still growing.

Now the realization may occur, possibly for the first time, that she could die, that her chances of surviving have been greatly reduced. Treatments for anything but a local recurrence are to "prolong life," not to cure a person. The doctors have already given the patient the latest and best combination of therapies. They did this believing that when the cancer comes back they don't have many options. Chemotherapy and radiation are used as the first line of defense, with greater success when the patient is in good overall health. A second or third course of these treatments can permanently weaken the immune system. With recurrence, the whole mood changes; even the doctors are less optimistic. The patient may sense this, no matter what reassuring words are used.

As a friend or family member, you will most certainly recognize this as another crisis. If the cancer can still be surgically removed, this is often considered the first course of action. For some women, alternative treatments seem more attractive once the standard medical approaches prove fallible. They may want to change their diet, start meditating, or go to Europe or Mexico for some special treatment that you have never heard of. This is another opportunity to offer your help. The exploration of all these options needs to be supported if her hope is to be maintained.

I think that often when women fail at alternative therapies, it is because some family member initiated a therapy and the woman only moderately supported the idea, or the woman investigates and finds something she believes in, but her family and friends discourage her and try to get her to return to conventional treatment. When a cancer patient eats all alone because she needs a special diet, then family and friends are not supporting her. Alternative therapies are not a punishment for having a recurrence; they are a gift, one I hope you can share with the person you love. I have never heard of someone getting sick because they improved their diet, for instance.

Alice Elaine Cler, an oncology nurse, writes in *Cancer, God and I and a Natural Cure*[1] that she decided on alternative treatments as soon as she heard her advanced-stage breast-cancer diagnosis because she had seen the outcome in the hospital many times over. Her daughter (and co-author), Barbara Cler Pendleton, who is also a nurse, supported Alice by doing everything her mother had to do. She wanted to assure the safety of the program and lend emotional support in a way that she could do only by having the same experience.

For the woman with cancer, finding friends who will support her choices can mean changing friends. The thought of adopting new lifestyle patterns may feel threatening to those family and friends who don't want to consider that their own lifestyle may cause them to get cancer too. Many of my old, dear friends pulled away from me because they wanted to "go on with their lives and not think about breast cancer." But if only more women in the past had been thinking and talking about breast cancer, perhaps more people would be aware of the causes, and fewer women would be facing this disease. I understand where my former friends are coming from, but denial hasn't solved the problem yet.

Recurrence—on the basis of the statistics—shouldn't be unexpected. With this second diagnosis, friends and family need to be especially supportive of doing whatever it takes to restore the immune system and rid the body of the cancer. Alternative treatments are not covered by insurance. One way you can support your loved one or your friend is to offer financial assistance. Pay for an acupuncture treatment, Oriental herbs, 714X, the airplane trip for treatment, or having her house cleaned. Help her to not lose her dignity, her friends, and the people she needs the most to make it through the second round of treatments. Most of all, be there. Don't desert the patient—she still needs your help.

When I returned home from surgery I was shocked to find that my friends were too busy to come by and visit. They felt comfortable enough talking to me on the phone, but they had excuses that kept them from coming over. It was pretty astonishing how "unavailable" everyone suddenly became. A week later, when I called a group meeting, they all came to visit and were delighted to see me looking cheerful and normal. These indirect messages keep cancer patients smiling over their hurt. Regrettably, not too many people are open to seeing what is behind the smile.

Once a woman has a recurrence this does not mean she will soon die. She may have several recurrences or go into remission for a long period. Breast cancer does not always follow a predictable path.

WHEN DEATH BECOMES A REAL POSSIBILITY

Just as the first and second phase require space and emotional support, this last phase also requires that the caregivers and other people supporting her give the woman permission to choose. She may be too tired to follow a special diet; having cancer is exhausting. The cancer and some of the treatments gradually eat away at a person's will to live. When this happens, if the people in her support system are still trying to cheer her on, pushing life at all costs, then the patient's feelings aren't being respected. The patient and helpers are out of sync. The woman with breast cancer must be the director of this play. No one else has that right. When she decides to resign herself after fighting for years or only months, then that time is the right time.

If you can, help her to feel that resigning isn't failing and that you accept her choice; her work on earth may now be complete and it may be time to move on to another plane, even if everyone will miss her terribly. When the people around the woman give her this permission, her death is less stressful and is allowed to happen in a gentler and more peaceful way. It doesn't have to be the horrible experience everyone associates with cancer. But when family members aren't ready to let her go, the patient struggles to survive and prolongs the pain and loss of dignity.

Listen and be present for the patient. Let her tell you what she wants. Many books and articles describe how women and their families find peace in this time of transition and share very special moments. Turning a patient over to the hospital—out of sight and out of mind—is not the way I would choose for myself and not, I imagine, what most people want. Still, it happens because so few people feel able to be part of this experience. Seek help for yourself so that you can support the people you love. Hospice is available to help patients be comfortable at home and to keep this experience gentle and personal. These are the support people who can help the family and friends too. Death is part of life; yet no one really wants to talk about it. No one wants to think about their own mortality.

There are no training courses to teach us how to make departing beautiful. But helping a friend or loved family member who has breast cancer can be so simple: Be present, be available, and be loving.

APPENDIX 3

Reducing Your Breast-Cancer Risk Factors

No one yet knows how to prevent breast cancer, but women can take some proactive measures that may help reduce their risk and minimize environmental and health factors that are suspected of contributing to the increased rates of breast cancer:

1. Participate in outdoor activities for one hour at least three times a week.
2. Add UVA (full spectrum) light to work and home environments wherever possible, to enhance melatonin production.
3. Lower fat and sugar in diet to a maximum of 15 percent of total calorie intake.
4. Increase intake of vegetables, particularly dark green vegetables like kale, collards, and cabbage-family vegetables.
5. Avoid all synethetic hormones: oral contraceptives, foods that contain DES or other hormone residues (such as meat, poultry, eggs, and dairy products), and estrogen-replacement therapies, including tamoxifen.
6. Maintain a regular exercise program for a minimum of forty-five minutes, four times a week.
7. Lower stress with professional therapy, meditation, yoga, career satisfaction, and loving, supportive relationships.

APPENDIX 4

A Patient's Bill of Rights*

Source: From *A Patient's Bill of Rights*. Chicago: American Hospital Association (AHA).

1. The patient has the right to considerate and respectful care.
2. The patient has the right to and is encouraged to obtain from physicians and other direct caregivers relevant, current, and understandable information concerning diagnosis, treatment, and prognosis.

   Except in emergencies when the patient lacks decision-making capacity and the need for treatment is urgent, the patient is entitled to the opportunity to discuss and request information related to the specific procedures and/or treatments, the risks involved, the possible length of recuperation, and the medically reasonable alternatives and their accompanying risks and benefits.

   Patients have the right to know the identity of physicians, nurses, and others involved in their care, as well as when those involved are students, residents, or other trainees. The patient also has the right to know the immediate and long-term financial implications of treatment choices, insofar as they are known.
3. The patient has the right to make decisions about the plan of care prior to and during the course of treatment and to refuse a recommended treatment or plan of care to the extent permitted by law and hospital policy and to be informed of the medical consequences of this action. In case of such refusal, the patient is entitled to other appropriate care and services that the hospital provides or

* These rights can be exercised on the patient's behalf by a designated surrogate or proxy decision maker if the patient lacks decision-making capacity, is legally incompetent, or is a minor.

transfer to another hospital. The hospital should notify patients of any policy that might affect choice within the institution.

4. The patient has the right to have an advance directive (such as a living will, health care proxy, or durable power of attorney for health care) concerning treatment or designating a surrogate decision maker with the expectation that the hospital will honor the intent of the directive to the extent possible by law and hospital policy.

   Health care institutions must advise patients of their rights under state law and hospital policy to make informed medical choices, ask if the patient has an advance directive, and include that information in patient records. The patient has the right to timely information about hospital policy that may limit its ability to implement fully a legally valid advance directive.

5. The patient has the right to every consideration to privacy. Case discussion, consultation, examination, and treatment should be conducted to protect each patient's privacy.

6. The patient has the right to expect that all communications and records pertaining to his/her care will be treated as confidential, except in cases such as suspected abuse and public health hazards when reporting is permitted or required by law. The patient has the right to expect that the hospital will emphasize the confidentiality of this information when it releases it to any other parties entitled to review information in these records.

7. The patient has the right to review the records pertaining to his/her medical care and to have the information explained or interpreted as necessary, except when restricted by law.

8. The patient has the right to expect that, within its capacity and policies, a hospital will make reasonable response to the request of a patient for appropriate and medically indicated care and services. The hospital must provide evaluation, service, and/or referral as indicated by the urgency of the case. When medically appropriate and legally permissible, or when a patient has so requested, a patient may be transferred to another facility. The institution to which the patient is to be transferred must first have accepted the patient for transfer. The patient must also have the benefit of complete information and explanation concerning the need for, risks, benefits, and alternatives to such a transfer.

9. The patient has the right to ask and be informed of the existence of business relationships among the hospital, educational institutions, other health care providers, or payers that may influence the patient's treatment and care.

10. The patient has the right to consent to or decline to participate in proposed research studies or human experimentation affecting care and treatment or requiring direct patient involvement and to have those studies fully explained prior to consent. A patient who declines to participate in research or experimentation is entitled to the most effective care that the hospital can otherwise provide.
11. The patient has the right to expect reasonable continuity of care when appropriate and to be informed by physicians and other caregivers of available and realistic patient care options when hospital care is no longer appropriate.
12. The patient has the right to be informed of hospital policies and practices that relate to patient care, treatment, and responsibilities. The patient has the right to be informed of available resources for resolving disputes, grievances, and conflicts, such as ethics committees, patient representatives, or other mechanisms available in the institution. The patient has the right to be informed of the hospital's charges for services and available payment methods.

The collaborative nature of health care requires that patients, or their families/surrogates, participate in their care. The effectiveness of care and patient satisfaction with the course of treatment depends, in part, on the patient fulfilling certain responsibilities. Patients are responsible for providing information about past illnesses, hospitalizations, medications, and other matters related to health status. To participate effectively in decision making, patients must be encouraged to take responsibility for requesting additional information or clarification about their health status or treatment when they do not fully understand information and instructions. Patients are also responsible for ensuring that the health care institution has a copy of their written advance directive if they have one. Patients are responsible for informing their physicians and other caregivers if they anticipate problems in following prescribed treatment.

Patients should also be aware of the hospital's obligations to be reasonably efficient and equitable in providing care to other patients and the community. The hospital's rules and regulatlons are designed to help the hospital meet this obligation. Patients and their families are responsible for making reasonable accommodations to the needs of the hospital, other patients, medical staff, and hospital employees. Patients are responsible for providing necessary claims and for working with the hospital to make payment arrangements, when necessary.

A person's health depends on much more than health care services. Patients are responsible for recognizing the impact of their lifestyle on their personal health.

CONCLUSION

Hospitals have many functions to perform, including the enhancement of health status, health promotion, and the prevention of injury and disease; the immediate and ongoing care and rehabilitation of patients; the education of health professionals, patients, and the community; and research. All these activities must be conducted with an overriding concern for the values and dignity of patients.

A Patient's Bill of Rights was first adopted by the American Hospital Association (AHA) in 1973. This revision was approved by the AHA Board of Trustees on October 21, 1992.

Endnotes

Introduction

1. When this text was originally written in 1991, this number was 142,000. After standing at 142,900 for some years it has now been revised by the American Cancer Society to this much higher estimate. What I've learned over time is how very fluid cancer statistics really are.

Chapter 1

1. Fritjof Capra, *The Tao of Physics: An Exploration of the Parallels Between Modern Physics and Eastern Mysticism* (New York: Bantam Books, 1977).

Chapter 2

1. Curtis Mettlin, "Breast Cancer Risk Factors: Contributions to Planning Breast Cancer Control," *Cancer* Supplement 69, no. 7 (April 1, 1992), 1904–10. Three tables from this article are given here: Personal Risk Factors for Breast Cancer, Environmental Risk Factors for Breast Cancer, and Factors Limiting the Application of Knowledge of Risk Factors to Breast Cancer Prevention
2. Susan M. Love, M.D., *Dr. Susan Love's Breast Book* (Reading, Mass.: Addison-Wesley, 1990), 137–51.
3. Women with six or more pregnancies showed lower risk. A full-term pregnancy is required to influence the epithelial cells in the breast. These cells are influenced by high levels of prolactin, estrogen, and progesterone, which decrease with age and full-term pregnancy. Recent studies on oral-contraceptive use suggest that full-term pregnancy at an even earlier age, younger than twenty years, is necessary to lower risk. A. Mellemgaard, et al., "The Association Between Risk of Breast Cancer and Age at First Pregnancy and Parity in Maribo County, Denmark," *Acta Oncologica* 29 (1990), 705–707.
4. The protective effect of breast-feeding continues to be a controversial issue; however, a recent study and review of the data suggest that a protective effect was highest in premenopausal women who lactated for seven to nine months. Keun-Young Yoo, et al., "Independent Protective Effect of Lactation Against Breast Cancer: A Case Control Study in Japan," *American Journal of Epidemiology* 35, no. 7 (1992), 726–33.
5. Love, *Breast Book,* 143–44.
6. Loraine H. Frost and Robert L. Jackson, "Growth and Development of Infants Receiving a Proprietary Preparation of Evaporated Milk with Dextri-maltose and Vitamin D," *Journal of Pediatrics* 39 (1951), 585–92.

7. Ibid., 586. Diluted cow's milk is shown as containing 2.8 percent protein, human milk 1.5 percent, and an evaporated milk dilution 2.8 percent.
8. Ibid., 586.
9. Kathy Kane, M.A., R.D., "Lactose Intollerance Is Not a Food Allergy," *Health Focus,* May 1990, Burlington Health Center.
10. Andis Robeznieks, "The Perfect Food? Not Everyone Agrees," *Vegetarian Times,* April 1987.
11. *GP,* November 1951, advertisement for Mull-Soy, The Borden Company, states, "almost a quarter million babies annually allergic to cow's milk . . . one of every fifteen infants."
12. John A. McDougall and Mary A. McDougall, *The McDougall Plan* (Piscataway, N.J.: New Century Publishers, 1983), 51.
13. Phenobarbital is a barbiturate listed in *Taber's Cyclopedic Medical Dictionary* as "used in treatment of epilepsy because it has a depressive effect on motor area of the cerebral cortex." The cerebral cortex is the area of the brain responsible for motor projections, receiving impulses from the sensory organs such as the eyes, ears, and nose. Phenobarbital perhaps caused or contributed to my damaged eye-brain coordination, resulting in my crossed eyes and diminished olfactory sense. The doctors always told me that my eyes crossed not because of a muscle problem but because of faulty coordination between my eyes and my brain. They were never able to explain what would cause this condition.
14. Rose E. Frisch, et al., "Lower Lifetime Occurrence of Breast Cancer and Cancers of the Reproductive System among Former College Atheletes," *American Journal of Clinical Nutrition* 45 (1987), 328–35.
15. Susan Love, M.D., Testimony to the United States Senate Subcommittee on Aging, Committee on Labor and Human Resources, June 20, 1991. Response to committee topic: *Why are We Losing the War on Breast Cancer?*
16. Love, *Breast Book,* 145.
17. Neal D. Barnard, M.D., "Women and Cancer: Opportunities for Prevention." Reprinted from *PCRM Update,* September/October 1991.
18. February 26, 1992, at the Harvard School of Public Health.
19. Sherwood Gorbach, et al., *The Doctor's Anti-Breast Cancer Diet* (New York: Simon and Schuster, 1984), 3.
20. A. Ekbom, et al., "Evidence of prenatal influences on breast cancer risk," *Lancet* (October 24, 1992), 1015–18.
21. "Statistics Verify Trend of More Women Giving Birth After Age 30," *Burlington Free Press,* 1 December 1989, dateline: Atlanta.
22. Natalee S. Greenfield, *"First Do No Harm . . . ": A Dying Woman's Battle Against the Physicians and Drug Companies Who Misled Her about the Hazards of The Pill* (New York: Sun River Press, Two Continents Publishing Group, 1976).
23. Joseph Highland, et al., *Malignant Neglect* (New York: Alfred A. Knopf, 1979), 184.
24. Package insert, Tri-Levelen 21, Bertex Laboratories, Inc., May 1990.
25. Kim Painter, "Report Says Birth Control Can Aid Women's Health." *Burlington Free Press,* 23 April 1991.
26. H. Olsson, "Oral Contraceptives and Breast Cancer," *Acta Oncologica* 28 (1989), 857.
27. Ibid., 853.
28. Ibid., 853.
29. Ibid., 851.
30. Ibid., 850–51.

31. Rose Kushner, *Alternatives: New Developments in the War on Breast Cancer* (New York: Warner Books, 1984), 128–50.
32. Ibid., 138.
33. Donald R. Miller, et al., "Breast Cancer Before Age 45 and Oral Contraceptive Use: New Findings," *American Journal of Epidemiology* (1989), 269–80.
34. C. E. D. Chilvers and J. M. Deacon, Editorial: "Oral Contraceptives and Breast Cancer," *British Journal of Cancer* 61 (1990), 1–4.
35. Joseph Highland, et al., *Malignant Neglact,* 184.
36. Dimitrios Trichopoulos, "Hypothesis: Does Breast Cancer Originate in Utero?" *Lancet* (April 21, 1990), 939–40.
37. DES is used today to treat disturbances of menopause; it is reported to be more potent than natural estrogen.
38. Gena Corea, *The Hidden Malpractice: How American Medicine Mistreats Women* (New York: Harper Colophon Books, 1985), 280.
39. John Robbins, *Diet for a New America* (Walpole, N.H.: Stillpoint, 1987), 312.
40. Ibid.
41. Joseph Highland, et al., *Malignant Neglect.*
42. Rose Kushner, *Alternatives,* 136.
43. Jane Brody, in a *New York Times* article, "From Fertility to Mood: Sunlight Found to Affect Human Biology," examines the work of research psychiatrist Alfred Lewy and professor of endocrinology and metabolism Richard J. Wurtman. Research psychiatrist Wayne P. London offers groundbreaking research in "Reversed Cerebral Asymmetry and Breast Cancer," *Lancet* (April 25, 1992), 1055–56. Richard Stevens in *The American Journal of Epidemiology* 125 (1987), 556–61, offers "Electric Power Use and Breast Cancer: A Hypothesis."
44. "Outer Limits: Electricity and Cancer," *Longevity,* June 1991.
45. Brody, "From Fertility to Mood."
46. "Searching for a Better Pill," *Newsweek,* 8 April 1991, 56.
47. Patricia McCormac, "The Role of Light in Human Health Given New Importance," *The Los Angeles Times,* 17 February 1980.
48. Ibid.
49. Ibid.
50. "Outer Limits: Electricity and Cancer," *Longevity,* June 1991.
51. Louis Slesin, "The Danger of Ignoring Non-Ionizing Radiation," *Technology Review,* 22 January 1989.
52. Tore Tynes and Aage Andersen, "Electromagnetic Fields and Male Breast Cancer," *Lancet* (December 22/29, 1990), 1596.
53. Genevieve M. Matanoski, Patrick N. Breysse, and Elizabeth A. Elliott, "Electromagnetic Field Exposure and Male Breast Cancer," *Lancet* (March 23, 1991), 737.
54. H. Olsson, 849.
55. Love, *Breast Book,* 161.
56. Daniel A. Hoffman, John E. Lonstein, Michele M. Morin, et al., "Breast Cancer in Women with Scoliosis Exposed to Multiple Diagnostic X-Rays," *Journal National Cancer Institute* (September 6, 1989), 1307–12.
57. Love, *Breast Book,* 162.
58. Virginia Soffa, "Mammogram Radiation Varies between Vermont Facilities," *Hospital News,* February 1991, 20, 25.
59. Diana Hunt, "Mammogram Alert," *East West Journal,* September/October 1991, 57.

60. Daniel Haney (AP), "Report Links Strong X-Rays with Breast Cancer," *Burlington Free Press,* 26 December 1991, A1–2.
61. *New York Times,* "Radiation Is Shown to Be Greater than Expected for Those Who Fly Often," 14 February 1990, A-18. The article reports that airline and association officials do not believe that radiation should be a priority issue. "In terms of actual known risk, the FAA has a lot more pressing problems," stated Dr. Donald E. Hudson, of the Air Line Pilots Association.

Chapter 3

1. Jerome Cohen, Joseph W. Cullen, and L. Robert Martin, *Psychosocial Aspects of Cancer* (New York: Raven Press, 1982), 230.
2. James T. Patterson, *The Dread Disease: Cancer and Modern American Culture* (Cambridge, Mass: Harvard University Press, 1987), 12.
3. L. J. Rather, *The Genesis of Cancer: A Study in the History of Ideas* (Baltimore: The Johns Hopkins University Press, 1978), 9–10.
4. Michael Baum, *Breast Cancer: The Facts* (New York: Oxford University Press, 1988), 1.
5. Donald Attwater, *The Penguin Dictionary of the Saints* 2nd ed. (New York: Penguin, 1983), 32.
6 John J. Delancey, *Dictionary of Saints* (Garden City, New York: Doubleday, 1980), 30.
7. Baum, 2.
8. Baum, 3.
9. Baum, 3.
10. Baum, 5.
11. Nodes perceptible by touch, above the collarbone at the base of the neck.
12. Baum, 4–6.
13. Baum, 4.
14. Baum, 6.
15. Baum, 58.
16. Baum, 59.
17. Baum, 60.
18. Baum, 60
19. J. Stjensward, "Decreased Survival Related to Irradiation Postoperatively in Early Operable Breast Cancer," *Lancet* (November 30, 1974), 1285–86.
20. Baum, 65–66.
21. Baum, 65.
22. Gina Kolata, "Breast Cancer Consensus," *Science,* 27 September 1985.
23. Mary Spletter, *A Woman's Choice: New Options in the Treatment of Breast Cancer* (Boston: Beacon Press, 1982), 126.
24. Spletter, 126.
25. David Schrieberg, "Mother's Breast," *Mother Jones,* November–December 1992, 38.
26. J. L. Haybittle, D. Brinkley, J. Houghton, et al., "Postoperative Radiotherapy and Late Mortality: Evidence from the Cancer Research Campaign Trial for Early Breast Cancer," *British Medical Journal* 298 (1989), 1611, 1613.
27. Bernard Fisher, et al., "The Contributions of Recent NSABP Clinical Trials of Primary Breast Cancer Therapy to an Understanding of Tumor Biology: An Overview of Findings," *Cancer* Supplement (August 1980), 1009–23.
28. Joseph Highland, et al., *Malignant Neglect* (New York: Alfred Knopf, 1979), 145–59.

29. C. R. Hamilton and R. B. Buchanan, "Radiotherapy for Ductal Carcinoma in Situ Detected by Screening," *British Medical Journal* 301 (28 July 1990), 224–25.
30. L. Solin, et al., "The Detection of Local Reccurence after Definitive Irradiation for Early Stage Carcinoma of the Breast," *Cancer* 11 (1990), 2497–2502.
31. Highland, et al., 156.
32. Jerry E. Bishop, "Study Links Breast Cancer Treatment to Higher Risk of the Disease in Lungs," *The Wall Street Journal,* 14 May 1993, B6.
33. Michael Baum, "Trends in Primary Breast Cancer Management: Where Are We Going?" *Surgical Clinics of North America* 70 (October 1990), 1187–92.
34. "Chemotherapy No Cure for Breast Cancer," *Vegetarian Times,* August 1990.
35. Marc L. Citron, *Cancer and Leukemia Group Memorandum, Activation of Protocol 9193* (22 March, 1991).
36. David A. Ginsburg, et al., "Systemic Adjuvant Therapy for Node-Negative Breast Cancer," *Journal of the American Medical Association* (11 April, 1990).
37. Citron.
38. N. Padmanabhan, et al., "Mechanism of Action of Adjuvant Chemotherapy in Early Breast Cancer," *Lancet* (23 August 1986), 411–14.
39. "Early Breast Cancer Trialists' Collaborative: Systemic Treatment of Early Breast Cancer by Hormonal, Cytotoxic, or Immune Therapy," *Lancet* (4 January 1992), 1–15; (11 January 1992), 71–85.
40. David L. Page, "Prognosis and Breast Cancer: Recognition of Lethal and Favorable Prognostic Types," *The American Journal of Surgical Pathology* 15 (1991), 334–49.

Chapter 4

1. Dan Millman, *Way of the Peaceful Warrior: A Book That Changes Lives* (Tiburon, Calif.: H. S. Kramer, Inc., 1984).

Chapter 5

1. Jeffrey Bland, Ph.D., "Cancer Prevention versus Cancer Treatment," in *Your Health Under Siege: Using Nutrition to Fight Back* (Brattleboro, Vt.: Stephen Greene Press, 1981).
2. T. Collin Campbell, Ph.D., et al., *Mortality Rates in Transition in the People's Republic of China* (unpublished, 1990).
3. T. McKeown and R. G. Record, "Reasons for the Decline in Mortality in England and Wales During the Twentieth Century," *Population Studies* 29 (1975), 391–422.
4. Frank Falck, Jr., et. al., "Pesticides and Polychlorinated Bi-phenyl Residues in Human Breast Lipids and Their Relation to Breast Cancer," *Archives of Environmental Health* 47 (March/April 1992), 143–146.
5. Jerome B. Westin and Elihu Richter, "The Israeli Breast-Cancer Anomoly," *Annals New York Academy of Sciences,* Vol. 609 Trends in Cancer Mortality in Industrial Countries, 1990.
6. Ibid.
7. "Blood Levels of Organochlorine Residues and Risk of Breast Cancer," *Journal of the National Cancer Institute* 85 (1993), 648–52.
8. Rachel Carson, *Silent Spring* (Boston: Houghton Mifflin, 1962).
9. Fruit and vegetable displays piled to the ceilings are also an extravagance that increases eye appeal—but also waste. Our waste becomes another country's famine. Consumers contribute to the imbalance in global food consumption when we buy into this kind of marketing.

10. Leonard Cohen, *Journal of the National Cancer Institute* (3 April 1991) as reported by the Associated Press in the *Burlington Free Press* on the same date.
11. Boyd S. Eaton, et. al., *The Paleolithic Prescription: A Program of Diet and Exercise and a Design for Living* (New York: Harper & Row, 1988), 7.
12. "Feeding Frenzy," *Newsweek,* 27 May 1991, 45–53.
13. "Prevention is the Next Frontier," *Vogue* (October 1990), 280–84, 280. Reference Jack Fishman, Professor of biochemistry and molecular biology, University of Miami Medical School.
14. Campbell et al., *Mortality Rates in Transition.*
15. Paolo Toniolo, et al., "Calorie-providing Nutrients and Risk of Breast Cancer," *Journal of the National Cancer Institute* 81 (February 15, 1989), 278—86.
16. Walter C. Willett, et al., "Dietary Fat and Fiber in Relation to Risk of Breast Cancer: An 8-year Follow-up," *Journal of the American Medical Association* 268 (1992), 2037–44.
17. Meera Jain, et al., "Canadian Study Affirms Link Between Breast Cancer and Fat Intake," *Journal of the National Cancer Institute* (March 6, 1991), *Boston Globe* report of above article.
18. "In spite of its high calcium content, milk, due to its high protein content, appears to actually *contribute* to the accelerating development of osteoporosis." John Robbins, *Diet For a New America.*
19. Frank Oski, M.D., *Don't Drink Your Milk,* (Mollica Press, 1983).
20. John A. McDougall, M.D., and Mary A. McDougall, *The McDougall Plan* (Piscataway, N.J.: New Century Publishers, 1983).
21. Susan M. Love, M.D., *Dr. Susan Love's Breast Book* (Reading, Mass.: Addison-Wesley, 1990), 81–87.
22. Lynn Rosenberg, Linda Metzger, and Julie Palmer, "Alcohol Consumption and Risk of Breast Cancer: A Review of the Epidemiologic Evidence," *Epidemiologic Reviews* vol. 5, 1993, 133–44.
23. Ibid., 141.
24. Kay W. Colston, et. al., "Possible Role for Vitamin D in Controlling Breast Cancer Cell Proliferation," *Lancet,* 28 January 1989, 188–91.
25. Noboru Muramoto, *Natural Immunity Insights on Diet and AIDS* (Oroville, Calif.: George Ohsawa Macrobiotic Foundation, 1988), 150.
26. Jane E. Brody, "Emotions Found to Influence Nearly Every Human Ailment," *New York Times,* 24 May 1983.

Chapter 6

1. Mary Spletter, *A Woman's Choice: New Options in the Treatment of Breast Cancer* (Boston: Beacon Press, 1982), 115–16.
2. Susan M. Love, M.D., with Karen Lindsey, *Dr. Love's Breast Book* (Reading, Mass.: Addison-Wesley, 1990).
3. R. Badwe, et al., "Timing of Surgery During Menstrual Cycle and Survival of Premenopausal Women with Operable Breast Cancer," *Lancet* 337 (25 May 1991) ,1261–64.
4. Patricia Bredenberg, *Who Cares? Women with Breast Cancer and Social Support* (Doctoral Dissertation, Syracuse University, Syracuse, New York, June 1991).
5. Ibid.
6. Ibid.
7. Douglas Marchant, M.D., Professor of OB/GYN and surgery at Tufts University of Medicine, Keynote Speaker, Maine Medical Center Annual Cancer Symposium: Breast Cancer, 17 May 1991, Portland, Maine.

8. For more information contact the American Society for Laser Medicine and Surgery, Inc., 2404 Stewart Square, Wausau, WI 54401, 715-845-9283.
9. "The Medical Breakthroughs Are Amazing–But Many Patients Never Get the Treatment," *Ladies Home Journal,* September 1991, 226.
10. Gina Kolata, "Breast Cancer Consensus," *Science* 229 (27 September 1985).
11. Richard Vernaci, "Experts describe breast-implant problems," as reported by the Associated Press in the *Burlington Free Press,* "Spotlight on Health" section, (19 February 1992).
12. George W. Mitchell, Jr., and Lawrence W. Bassett, *The Female Breast and Its Disorders* (Baltimore: Williams & Wilkins,1990), 232 (refers to R. E. Wilson, "Progress in Breast Cancer Treatment, Today and Tomorrow," *American College Surgical Bulletin,* 68:2 (1983). A recent Canadian study indicates 80 percent of the operations performed are still mastectomies. And a 1982 audit in the U.S. indicates that "at least 80 percent of all patients undergoing surgical treatment for breast cancer have the modified radical procedure."
13. Bernard Fisher, et al., "Five-year Results of a Randomized Clinical Trial Comparing Total Mastectomy and Segmental Mastectomy With or Without Radiation in the Treatment of Cancer," *New England Journal of Medicine* 312 (1985), 665–73; "Eight-year Results," *New England Journal of Medicine* 320 (1989), 822–28.

Chapter 7

1. Richard Hittleman, *Yoga: 28-Day Exercise Plan* (New York: Bantam Books, 1969).
2. Saskia R. J. Thiadens, R.N., Thom W. Rooke, M.D., and John P. Cooke, M.D., Ph.D., F.A.C.C., "Lymphedema," *Current Management of Hypertensive and Vascular Disease* (1991), 314–19.
3. Norman Cousins, *Anatomy of An Illness* (New York: W. W. Norton, 1979).
4. Arnold Fox, M.D., and Barry Fox, Ph.D., "Keeping Your Immune System Strong," *Let's Live* (August 1989).
5. "Green Tea Could Help Prevent Cancer, Research Shows," *Burlington Free Press,* 27 August 1991.
6. A free radical is defined as any molecule that has an unpaired electron in its outer orbit. When a molecule loses one of its electrons, it becomes highly reactive and imbalanced. Excess free radicals are a direct result of the chemical, emotional, physical, and infectious stresses we encounter.
7. Press Release PR Newswire Assoc., Inc., 13 May 1993.
8. Christopher Bird, *The Persecution and Trial of Gaston Naessens* (Tiburon, Calif.: H. J. Kramer Inc., 1991).

Chapter 8

1. Joan Borysenko, Ph.D., *Minding the Body, Mending the Mind* (New York: Bantam Books, 1988), 21.
2. Carol S. Pearson, *The Hero Within* (San Francisco: Harper & Row, 1986, 1989), 84.
3. Carlos Castaneda, *The Teaching of Don Juan* (New York: Pocket Books, 1972).
4. I. Jaiyesimi and A. Buzdar, et al. "Carcinoma of the Male Breast," *Annals of Internal Medicine* (vol. 117, 1992), 771–77.
5. John Bailar and Elaine M. Smith, "Progress Against Cancer," *New England Journal of Medicine* (May 1986), 1226–32.
6. Sharon Batt, "Cancer Victims Can Learn from AIDS Sufferers," *The Gazette Canada* (4 July 1989).

7. David Spiegel, "Breast Cancer Study Shows Psychotherapy Improved Survival," *Psychiatric Times* (January 1990). "Our research team was shocked to find that, on average, members of a group of 86 women with metastatic breast cancer who received psychotherapy . . . lived twice as long as those in the control group. Those assigned to psychotherapy attended weekly support group sessions for a year. The control group received oncological treatment but no psychotherapy."
8. Patricia Bredenberg, Ph.D., R.N., "Who Cares? Women with Breast Cancer and Social Support," a talk at the Annual Symposium on Breast Cancer, Maine Medical Center, Portland, Maine, 17 May 1991.
9. Ibid.
10. Ibid.

Chapter 9

1. Feminist Majority Foundation, *Empowering Women in Medicine,* 1991.
2. Testifying before the House Appropriations Subcommittee on Labor, Health and Human Services and Education in March 1992, Dr. Healy declared that although she is a strong supporter of research on women's health, she opposes such an earmark. "It would be destructive . . . to have $500 million earmarked specifically for women's health," she stated. Reference: *Update: On Women and Family Issues In Congress,* Vol. 12 No. 2, March 31, 1992, prepared by the Congressional Caucus for Women's Issues. In May 1992, Dr. Healy sent a letter to Dr. Louis Sullivan, Secretary of Health, recommending that if Congress approves the above earmarked dollars, the President veto this legislation.
3. Ruth Hubbard, *The Politics of Women's Biology* (New Brunswick, N.J.: Rutgers University Press, 1990), 37.
4. Ibid., 27.
5. Ibid., 38.
6. A newly formed President's Cancer Panel: A Special Commission on Breast Cancer, carefully selected an equal number of women commissioners; however, the majority of them are scientific professionals who have resisted any public declaration of their personal experience with breast cancer. This, the NCI states, would be a violation of their medical history.
7. Ruth Hubbard, 32.
8. Rose Kushner, *Alternatives: New Developments in the War on Breast Cancer* (New York: Warner Books, 1984), 128-50.
9. U.S. General Accounting Office (GAO), report (1990) from Congress' investigative agency, which found that there is an "under representation of women" in federally funded studies. This report inspired the introduction of the Health Equity Act by Rep. Patricia Schroeder (D-Colo.) and the creation of the Office for Women's Health Research under the Director of the NIH.
10. Margaret Lock, "Contested Meanings of Menopause," *Lancet* (25 May 1991), 127–72.
11. K.-Y. Yoo, K. Tajima, et al., "Independent Protective Effect of Lactation Against Breast Cancer: A Case-Control Study in Japan," *American Journal of Epidemiology 135 (1992), 726–33.*
12. J. L. Kelsey, and M. D. Gammon, "Epidemiology of Breast Cancer," *Epidemiologic Review* 12 (1990), 228–40.
13. Lock, "Contested Meanings of Menopause," 1270–72.
14. In the early 1980s, a lobbying group called the American Society of Plastic and Reconstructive Surgeons, Inc., issued a memo to the FDA asserting, "There is a substantial and enlarging body of medical information and opinion to the effect that

these deformities [small breasts] are really a disease that, left uncorrected, results in a total lack of well-being." This same group has spent vast sums of money to persuade government agencies that breast implants are a safe way to "correct" such "diseases." See the next chapter, "The Politics of Breast Cancer."

15. Gena Corea, *The Hidden Malpractice* (New York: Harper Colophon Books, 1985), 171.
16. *Ca: A Cancer Journal for Clinicians* 41 (January–February 1991), 23.
17. The Breast and Cervical Cancer Prevention Act founded by Congress beginning in 1990 focuses on the needs of "poor and underserved" women.
18. A. D. G. Gunn, *Oral Contraception in Perspective: Thirty years of clinical experience with the pill* (Fort Myers, Fla.: Parthenon Publishing Group, 1987).
19. "Lower Dose Pills," *Population Reports*, November 1988 Series A, No. 7.
20. Kushner, *Alternatives,* 128–50.
21. Kushner, *Alternatives*, 129.
22. *Population Reports.*
23. *Population Reports.*
24. Ibid.
25. P. N. Matthews, et al., "Breast Cancer in Women Who Have Taken Contraceptive Steroids," *British Medical Journal* 282 (1981), 774.
26. "Lopsided Drug Ads Mislead Doctors, Researchers Say," *Los Angeles Times,* (1 June, 1992) reference study lead author Michael S. Wilkes, a UCLA professor of medicine.
27. Premarin, a conjugated estrogen tablet produced by Wyeth-Amerst Laboratories, has been distributed since the 1950s.
28. Alisa Solomon, "The Politics of Breast Cancer: Refusing to let the disease remain a private burden, new cancer activists are talking about a revolution," *The Village Voice* (14 May 1991).
29. Elizabeth Neus, "Study: Battered Women Like Hostages,"*Burlington Free Press* (17 August 1991).

Chapter 10

1. Joe Thornton, "Breast Cancer and the Environment: The Chlorine Connection," Greenpeace report (1992), 19–20.
2. American Cancer Society, Professional Education Publication, *Guidelines for the Cancer-Related Checkup: Recommendations and Rationale, Ca: A Cancer Journal for Clinicians* 30, no. 4 (1980).
3. Ibid.
4. John Cassidy and Tim Rayment, "Women Who Have Breast Scanning Are More Likely to Die of Cancer," *The Sunday Times,* 2 June 1991.
5. Quentin J. Walker, et al., "The Misuse of Mammography in the Management of Breast Cancer Revisited," *JAMA* 263 (1990), 1980–81.
6. David M. Eddy, et al., "The Value of Mammography Screening in Women Under Age 50 Years," *JAMA* 259 (1988), 1512–19.
7. Peter Skrabanek, "Screening for Disease: False Premises and False Promises of Breast Cancer Screening," *Lancet* (10 August 1985), 316–19.
8. United States General Accounting Office Report to Congressional Committees for January 1990, entitled *Screening Mammography, 1990.*
9. Virginia Soffa, "Mammogram Radiation Varies between Vermont Facilities," *Hospital News* (February 1991), 20.

10 Jacob Shapiro, *Radiation Protection: A Guide For Scientists and Physicians* (Cambridge: Harvard University Press, 1990), 94.

11. American Cancer Society, *Guidelines for the Cancer-Related Checkup* (1980), 36.

12. In 1990, Congress made into law the Breast and Cervical Cancer Screening Prevention Act to allocate $50 million for three consecutive years to the states for promotion and education of screening. This program is overseen by the Centers for Disease Control. Breast cancer receives a larger proportion than does cervical cancer. The 1993 budget received 70 million dollars.

13. High-risk is defined in the approved study guidelines, NCI, as follows: age 35 with one or more first-degree relatives with breast cancer, and the presence of benign breast disease found in at least two biopsies; age 40 with two or more first-degree relatives with cancer; age 45 or older with one or more first-degree relatives with breast cancer; age 55 with first live birth at age 30 or older; age 35 or older with the diagnosis of lobular carcinoma *in situ*.

14. David C. G. Skegg, "Potential for Bias in Case-Control Studies of Oral Contraceptives and Breast Cancer," *American Journal of Epidemiology* 127 (February 1988), 209.

15. American Cancer Society, *Guidelines for the Cancer-Related Checkup* (1980), 46.

16. Skegg, "Potential for Bias," 210.

17. Lisa Davis, "Breast Implants: Two Million Guinea Pigs?" *In Health* (September/October 1991), 30–34.

18. National Cancer Institute Breast Cancer Budget July 2, 1991.

19. The Congressional Budget for Fiscal Year 1993, Table 6–9. The budget proposes a 13 percent increase in federal funding for HIV and AIDS.

20. "Activists Fear AIDS Will Disappear from Public Agenda," *Burlington Free Press* (30 September 1991).

21. American Cancer Society Actual breast cancer deaths through 1988. National Cancer Insititute SEER 1989.

22. "AIDS Bill Tops $5 Billion in U.S., Study Estimates," *Burlington Free Press* (29 November 1991).

23. David Eddy, et al., "The Value of Mammography Screening," *JAMA* 259 (11 March 1988), 1512–19.

24. American Cancer Society, *Guidelines for the Cancer Related Checkup: Recommendations and Rational* (1980), 38.

25. Alisa Solomon, "The Politics of Breast Cancer," *The Village Voice* (14 May 1991), 26.

26. Ibid.

27. Ibid.

28. *Ladies Home Journal* (September 1991), 228.

29. Audre Lord, *The Cancer Journals* (San Francisco: Spinsters/Aunt Lute, 1980), 16.

Appendix 2

1. Alice Elaine Cler and Barbara Cler Pendleton, *Cancer God and I and a Natural Cure* (New York: Vantage Press, 1987).

Resources

The artwork in this book is part of the "Healing Legacies" slide registry. New artwork can be submitted to the Breast Cancer Action Group, P.O. Box 5605, Burlington, VT 05402.

BREAST CANCER ORGANIZATIONS

American Cancer Society &
Reach to Recovery
Data Base Hotline
1-800-ACS-2345

National Breast Cancer Coalition
P.O. Box 66373
Washington, DC 20035

National Cancer Institute
Information Hotline
1-800-422-6237

National Lymphedema Network, Inc.
221 Post Street, Suite 404
San Francisco, CA 94115

National Women's Health Network
1325 G Street NW
Washington, DC 20005
202-347-1140

Y-Me National Organization for Breast Cancer Information and Support
212 W. Van Buren
Chicago, IL 60607
1-800-221-2141

International

Breast Cancer Action Montreal
257 Villeneuve W. #5
Montreal, QUE H2V 2R2
Canada

The Alliance of Breast Cancer Survivors
20 Eglington Ave. W. Suite 1106
Toronto, ONT M4R 1K8
Canada

Burlington Breast Cancer Support Services
2nd. Floor Burlington Mall
777 Guelph Line
Burlington, ONT L7R 3N2
Canada

Canadian Breast Cancer Foundation
620 University Avenue Suite 702
Toronto, ONT M5G 2C1
Canada

Breast Cancer Reasearch & Education Fund
8 Pearl Ann Drive
St. Catharines, ONT L2T 3B3
Canada

Breast Care and Matectomy Association
15-19 Britten Street
London, SW3 3TZ
England

EDUCATIONAL RESOURCES

American Society of Dowsers
Danville, VT 05828
802-684-3417

Interface
55 Wheeler Street
Cambridge, MA 02138
617-876-4600

Kripalu Yoga and Health Center
P.O. Box 793
Lenox, MA 01240
413-448-3400

Kushi Institute
P.O. Box 8
Becket, MA 01223
413-623-5742

The Natural Gourmet Cookery School
48 West 21st Street, 2nd Floor
New York, NY 10010
212-645-5170

Omega Institute for Holistic Studies
260 Lake Drive
Rhinebeck, NY 12572
1-800-944-1001

The Open Center
83 Spring Street
New York, NY 10012
212-219-2527

Phoenix Rising Yoga Therapy
To obtain the number of a therapist in your area
1-800-288-9642

International

The Findhorn Foundation
Cluny Hill College
Forres IV 36 ORD
Scotland

Women's Health Information and Support Centre
Junction 7
3-7 Hazelwood Road
Northampton, NN1 1LG
England

Winsford Well Women's Information Centre
Wharton Clinic
Bradbury Road
Winsford, Cheshire CW 7
England

Meaningful Life Therapy
Shibata Hospital
6108 Tamashima—Otoshima
Kurashiki, 713
Japan

The Australian Cancer Patient's Foundation, Inc.
The Melbourne Living Center
360 Mont Albert Road
Mont Albert, Victoria 3127
Australia

The Yarra Living Center
P.O. Box 77
Yarra Junction
Australia

WOMEN'S/CANCER/ ENVIRONMENTAL ORGANIZATIONS

Women's Environment & Development Organization (WEDO)
845 Third Avenue, 15 Floor
New York, NY 10022
212-759-7982

Pesticide Action Network
116 New Montgomery Street Suite 810
San Francisco, CA 94105
415-541-9140

Foundation for a Compassionate Society
227 Congress Avenue
Austin, TX 78701-4201
512-472-0131

International

Women's Environmental Network
391 Cunningham Avenue
Ottawa, ONT K1H 6B3
Canada

International Institute of Concern for Public Health
830 Bathurst Street
Toronto, ONT M5R 3G1
Canada

Women and Environments Education and Development (WEED) Foundation
736 Bathurst Street
Toronto, ONT M5S 2R4
Canada

Women on the Move Against Cancer
c/o Burson—Marsteller
24-38 Bloomsbury Way
London, WC1A 2PX
England

Women's Nationwide Cancer Control Campaign
Suna House
128 Curtain Road
London, EC3A 3AR
England

Women's Environmental Network
Aberden Studios
22 Highbury Grove
London, N52EA
England

Fertility Action
P.O. Box 4569
Auckland, New Zealand

Women and Health
Women's Center Osaka
1-3-23 Gamo Joto-ku
Osaka, 536
Japan

Pesticide Action Network
P.O. Box 1170
10850 Penang
Malaysia

Carribean Women's Cancer Network
WAND, School of Continuing Studies
University of the West Indies
Pinelands, St. Michael
Barbados

Peruvian Women's Center
Flora Tristan
Parque Hernan Velarde 42
Lima, 1
Peru

Latin American & Carribean Women's Health Network
ISIS Internacional
Casilla 2067, Correo Central
Santiago
Chile

LISTSERV EMAIL DISCUSSION LISTS RELEVANT TO BREAST CANCER

The Cancer Liaison and Action Network discussion list
Listserv Name: clan
BITNET address: listserv@frmop11
Internet address: listserv@frmop11.cnusc.fr

The Women's Health Issues discussion list
Listserv Name: wmn-hlth
BITNET address: listserv@uwavm
Internet address: listserv@uwavm.u.washington.edu

The WVNET Cancer discussion list
Listserv Name: cancer-1
BITNET address: listserv@wvnvm
Internet address: listserv@wvnvm.wvnet.edu

IMPLANT NETWORKS/INFORMATION

Command Trust
P.O. Box 17082
Covington, KY 41017
606-331-0055

Global Settlement Information
(Class Action Suit)
1-800-887-6828

Impact
P.O. Box 16097
Oakland, CA 94610-9991
(Education, support & advocacy newsletter for women with problem implants)

MAIL ORDER FOOD, BOOKS, AND SUPPLIES

The Mail Order Catalog
P.O. Box 180
Summertown, TN 38483
1-800-695-2241

Super Blue-Green™ Algae
Cell Tech
1300 Main Street
Klamath Falls, OR 97601
1-800-800-1300

Mountain Ark Trader
120 South East Avenue
Fayetteville, AR 72701
1-800-643-8909

Water Filter
Multi-Pure Corporation
21339 Nordhoff Street
Chatsworth, CA 91311
1-800-622-9206

Local resources can be located through the Yellow Pages under headings of Health Food Stores, Consumer Cooperative Organizations (Co-Ops), and Restaurants–Vegetarian.

The local health food stores often have bulletin boards and personnel who are familiar with support groups, classes, practitioners, and restaurants in their area. When I travel I utilize these resources and have never been disappointed. When traveling by air you can request 24 hours in advance a vegetarian meal. Some airlines now offer a Vegetarian Non-Dairy option.

Suggested Reading List

BREAST CANCER AND CANCER BOOKS

Baum, Michael. *Breast Cancer: The Facts.* New York: Oxford University Press, 1988.

Bird, Christopher. *The Persecution and Trial of Gaston Naessens.* Tiburon, Calif.: H. J. Kramer Inc., 1991.

Brady, Judith, ed. *1 in 3 Women with Cancer Confront an Epidemic.* Pittsburgh: Cleiss Press, Inc., 1991.

Butler, Sandra, and Barbara Rosenblum. *Cancer in Two Voices.* San Francisco: Spinsters Books, 1991.

Cler, Alice Elaine, and Barbara Cler Pendleton. *Cancer God and I and a Natural Cure.* New York: Vantage Press, 1987.

Greenfield, Natalee S. *"First Do No Harm . . . ": A Dying Woman's Battle Against the Physicians and Drug Companies Who Misled Her about the Hazards of The Pill.* New York: Sun River Press, Two Continents Publishing Group, 1976.

Highland, Joseph, et al. *Malignant Neglect.* New York: Alfred A. Knopf, 1979.

Hirshaut, Yashar, and Peter Pressman. *Breast Cancer: The Complete Guide.* New York: Bantam Books, 1992.

Kahane, Deborah. *No Less a Woman: Ten Women Shatter the Myths about Breast Cancer.* New York: Prentice Hall, 1990.

Kaye, Ronnie. *Spinning Straw Into Gold: Your Emotional Recovery From Breast Cancer.* New York: Simon and Schuster, Inc., 1991.

Kushner, Harold S. *When Bad Things Happen to Good People.* New York: Schocken Books, 1981.

Kushner, Rose. *Alternatives: New Developments in the War on Breast Cancer.* New York: Warner Books, 1984.

Lord, Audre. *The Cancer Journals.* San Francisco: Spinsters/Aunt Lute, 1980.

Love, Susan M., M.D. *Dr. Susan Love's Breast Book.* Reading, Mass.: Addison-Wesley, 1990.

Mayer, Musa. *Examining Myself: One Woman's Story of Breast Cancer Treatment and Recovery.* Boston: Faber & Faber, 1993.

McDougall, John A. *McDougall's Medicine, A Challenging Second Opinion.* Piscataway, N.J.: New Century Publishers, Inc., 1983.

Nessim, Susan, and Judith Ellis. *Cancervive.* Boston: Houghton Mifflin, 1991.

Patterson, James T. *The Dread Disease: Cancer and Modern American Culture.* Cambridge, Mass: Harvard University Press, 1987.

Rather, L. J. *The Genesis of Cancer: A Study in the History of Ideas.* Baltimore: The Johns Hopkins University Press, 1978.

Rinzler, Carol Ann. *Estrogen and Breast Cancer.* New York: Macmillan, 1993.

Spletter, Mary. *A Woman's Choice: New Options in the Treatment of Breast Cancer.* Boston: Beacon Press, 1982.

Stocker, Midge, ed. *Cancer as a Woman's Issue.* Chicago: Third Side Press, 1991.

———. *Confronting Cancer, Constructing Change: New Perspectives on Women and Cancer.* Chicago: Third Side Press, 1993.

DIETS THAT HEAL

Barnard, Neal, M.D. *The Power of Your Plate.* Summertown, Tenn.: Book Publishing Co., 1990.

Colbin, Annemarie. *The Natural Gourmet.* New York: Ballantine Books, 1989.

Crook, William G., M.D. *The Yeast Connection: A Medical Breakthrough.* Jackson, Tenn.: Professional Books/Future Health, 1986.

Dufty, William. *Sugar Blues.* New York: Warner Books, 1975.

Erasmus, Udo. *Fats and Oils: The Complete Guide to Fats and Oils in Health and Nutrition.* Vancover: Alive, 1986.

Garland, Cedric, M.D., and Frank Garland, M.D. *The Calcium Connection.* New York: Putnam, 1988.

Kushi, Micho. *The Cancer Prevention Diet.* New York: St. Martin's Press, 1983.

McDougall, John A., M.D., and Mary A. McDougall. *The McDougall Plan.* Piscataway, N.J.: New Century Publishers, 1983.

Sattilaro, Anthony J., M.D. *Recalled by Life.* Avon Books, 1982.

Stewart, John Cary. *Drinking Water Hazards.* Hiram, Ohio: Envirographics, 1990.

ENLIGHTENED POEMS AND STORIES

Harper, Elizabeth Roberts. *Earth Prayers From Around the World.* San Francisco: Harper San Francisco, 1991.

Jones, Gladys V. *The Flowering Tree: A Mystical Interpretation of Reincarnation.* Marina del Ray, Calif.: DeVorss & Company, 1984.

Millman, Dan. *Way of the Peaceful Warrior: A Book That Changes Lives.* Tiburon, Calif.: H. S. Kramer, Inc., 1984.

FEMINISM AND PSYCHOLOGY

Benjamin, Jessica. *The Bonds of Love: Psychoanalysis, Feminism and the Problem of Domination.* New Jersey: Pantheon, 1988.

Borysenko, Joan, Ph.D. *Minding the Body, Mending the Mind.* New York: Bantam Books, 1988.

Chodorow, Nancy. *Feminism and Psychoanalytic Theory.* New Haven, Conn.: Yale University Press, 1989.

McWilliams, Peter, and John-Rodger McWilliams. *You Can't Afford the Luxury of a Negative Thought: A Book for People with Any Life-Threatening Illness—Including Life.* Los Angeles: Prelude Press, 1988.

Pearson, Carol S. *The Hero Within.* San Francisco: Harper & Row, 1986, 1989.

Pelletier, Kenneth. *Mind as Healer, Mind as Slayer.* New York: Dell Publishing Co., 1977.

Siegel, Elaine V., ed. *Psychoanalytic Perspectives on Women.* New York: Brunner/Mazel, 1992.

FOOD AND HEALTH

Carson, Rachel. *Silent Spring.* Boston: Houghton Mifflin, 1962.

Colbin, Annemarie. *The Book of Whole Meals.* New York: Ballantine Books, 1979.

———. *Food and Healing.* New York: Ballantine Books, 1986.

Eaton, Boyd S., M.D., et al. *The Paleolithic Prescription: A Program of Diet and Exercise and a Design for Living.* New York: Harper & Row, 1988.

McDougall, John A., M.D. and Mary A. McDougall. *The McDougall Plan.* Piscataway, N.J.: New Century Publishers, Inc., 1983.

Muramoto, Norboru. *Natural Immunity Insights on Diet and AIDS.* Oroville, Calif.: George Ohsawa Macrobiotic Foundation, 1988.

Ornstein, Robert, Ph.D., and David Sobel, M.D., *Healthy Pleasures.* Reading, Mass.: Addison-Wesley, 1989.

Robbins, John. *Diet for a New America.* Walpole, N.H.: Stillpoint, 1987.

Vegetarian Times. *Guide to Natural Food Restaurants in the U.S. and Canada.* Summertown, Tenn.: The Book Publishing Co., 1989.

Winter, Ruth. *A Consumers's Dictionary of Food Additives.* New York: Crown Publisher, 1989.

HEALING ARTS

Dackman, Linda. *Affirmations, Meditations, Encouragements for Women Living with Breast Cancer.* Los Angeles: Lowell House, 1991.

Desai, Yogi Amrit. *Kripalu Yoga: Meditation-In-Motion Book II: Focusing Inward.* Mass: Kripalu Yoga Fellowship, 1992.

Dreifuss-Kattan, Esther. *Cancer Stories: Creativity and Self-Repair.* Hillsdale, N.J.: Analytic Press, 1990.

Hanh, Thich Nhat. *Peace Is Every Step: The Path of Mindfulness in Everyday Life.* New York: Bantam Books, 1992.

Hittleman, Richard. *Richard Hittleman's Yoga.* New York: Bantam Books, 1969.

———. *Yoga: 28-Day Exercise Plan.* New York: Bantam Books, 1969.

Kornfield, Jack. *A Path with Heart: A Guide Through the Perils and Promises of Spiritual Life.* New York: Bantam Books, 1993.

LeShan, Lawrence. *How to Meditate.* New York: Bantam Books, 1974.

Rico, Gabriele. *Pain and Possibility: Writing Your Way Through Personal Crisis.* Los Angeles: Jeremy P. Tarcher, Inc., 1991.

Rodegast, Pat, and Stanton, Judith. *Emmanuel's Book: A Manual for Living Comfortably in the Cosmos.* New York: Bantam Books, 1987.

Rossman, Martin L. *Healing Yourself: A Step-by-Step Program for Better Health Through Imagery.* New York: Pocket Books, 1987.

Samuels, Mike, and Nancy Samuels. *Seeing With the Mind's Eye.* New York: Random House, 1975.

Weiss, Brian L. *Many Lives, Many Masters.* New York: Simon & Schuster, 1988.

HEALING JOURNEYS

Andrews, Lynn V. *Medicine Woman.* NewYork: Harper & Row, 1981.

Baker, Nancy C. *Relative Risk.* New York: Viking Penguin Books, 1991.

Broyard, Anatole. *Intoxicated by My Illness.* New York: Clarkson Potter, 1992.

Cousins, Norman. *Anatomy of an Illness.* New York: W.W. Norton & Co., 1979.

———. *Head First: The Biology of Hope.* New York: E. P. Dutton, 1989.

———. *The Healing Heart.* New York: Norton, 1983.

Kubler-Ross, Elisabeth. *On Death and Dying.* New York: Macmillan, 1969.

LeShan, Lawrence. *Cancer as a Turning Point.* New York: Dutton, 1989.

Levine, Stephen. *Healing into Life and Death: Where Is Healing to Be Found?* New York: Doubleday, 1987.

———. *Who Dies? An Investigation of Conscious Living and Conscious Dying.* New York: Doubleday, 1982.

Millman, Dan. *Way of the Peaceful Warrior.* Tiburon, Calif.: H. J. Kramer, Inc., 1984.

Moody, Raymond A. *Life After Life.* New York: Bantam Books, 1976.

Peck, M. Scott. *The Road Less Traveled.* New York: Simon and Schuster, 1978.

Siegel, Bernie S. *Love, Medicine and Miracles.* New York: Harper & Row, 1986.

———. *Peace, Love and Healing.* New York: Harper & Row, 1989.

Weiss, Brian L. *Through Time Into Healing.* New York: Simon & Schuster, 1992.

HEALTH SUPPORTING RECIPES

Colbin, Annemarie. *The Natural Gourmet.* New York: Ballantine Books, 1989.

———. *The Book of Whole Meals.* New York: Ballantine Books, 1983.

Edwards, Linda. *Baking for Health: Whole Food Baking for Better Health.* Garden City Park, N.Y.: Avery Publishing Group, 1988.

Kushi, Aveline, and Alex Jack. *Aveline Kushi's Complete Guide to Macrobiotic Cooking.* New York: Warner Books, 1985.

Lerman, Andrea Bliss. *The Macrobiotic Community Cookbook.* Garden City Park, N.Y.: Avery Publishing Group, 1989.

McCarty, Meredith. *American Macrobiotic Cuisine.* Eureka, Calif.: Turning Point Publishing, 1986.

Michell, Keith. *Practically Macrobiotic.* Rochester, Vt.: Healing Arts Press, 1988.

Quigley, Delia, and Polly Pitchford. *Starting Over: Learning to Cook with Natural Foods.* Summertown, Tenn.: Book Publishing Co., 1988.

WOMEN AND HEALTH CARE

Corea, Gena. *The Hidden Malpractice: How American Medicine Mistreats Women.* New York: Harper Colophon Books, 1985.

Ehrenreich, Barbara. *Complaints and Disorders: The Sexual Politics of Sickness.* New York: The Feminist Press, 1974.

Ehrenreich, Barbara, and Diedre English. *For Her Own Good: 150 Years of the Experts' Advice to Women.* Garden City, N.Y.: Anchor Press/Doubleday, 1978.

Fisher, Sue. *In the Patient's Best Interest: Women and the Politics of Medical Decisions.* New Brunswick, N.J.: Rutgers University Press, 1990.

Index